NEUROSCIENCE RESEARCH PROGRESS

# UNDERSTANDING CHILDREN WITH AUTISM SPECTRUM DISORDERS

# NEUROSCIENCE RESEARCH PROGRESS

Additional books and e-books in this series can be found on Nova's website under the Series tab.

NEUROSCIENCE RESEARCH PROGRESS

# UNDERSTANDING CHILDREN WITH AUTISM SPECTRUM DISORDERS

ANNE BOURQUE
EDITOR

nova
Medicine & Health
New York

## NOTICE TO THE READER

The Publisher has taken reasonable care in the preparation of this book, but makes no expressed or implied warranty of any kind and assumes no responsibility for any errors or omissions. No liability is assumed for incidental or consequential damages in connection with or arising out of information contained in this book. The Publisher shall not be liable for any special, consequential, or exemplary damages resulting, in whole or in part, from the readers' use of, or reliance upon, this material. Any parts of this book based on government reports are so indicated and copyright is claimed for those parts to the extent applicable to compilations of such works.

Independent verification should be sought for any data, advice or recommendations contained in this book. In addition, no responsibility is assumed by the Publisher for any injury and/or damage to persons or property arising from any methods, products, instructions, ideas or otherwise contained in this publication.

This publication is designed to provide accurate and authoritative information with regard to the subject matter covered herein. It is sold with the clear understanding that the Publisher is not engaged in rendering legal or any other professional services. If legal or any other expert assistance is required, the services of a competent person should be sought. FROM A DECLARATION OF PARTICIPANTS JOINTLY ADOPTED BY A COMMITTEE OF THE AMERICAN BAR ASSOCIATION AND A COMMITTEE OF PUBLISHERS.

Additional color graphics may be available in the e-book version of this book.

**Library of Congress Cataloging-in-Publication Data**

ISBN: 978-1-53617-647-6

*Published by Nova Science Publishers, Inc. † New York*

# CONTENTS

# PREFACE

*Understanding Children with Autism Spectrum Disorders* first discusses auditory processing disorders are, specifically how auditory processing problems can affect children with autism spectrum disorders, and appropriate evidence-based treatments.

The authors highlight the challenges associated with making a dual diagnosis, and discuss specific anatomical differences in the central auditory pathway and brain.

Also highlighted is the need for improved research on intervention programs and the important service needs for families and children with autism spectrum disorders.

A study is presented wherein pediatric volition among children with autism spectrum disorders participating in the Holland Bloorview (HB) FIRST® robotics program is measured.

A review is carried out in order to describe the main neurotransmitters in autism spectrum condition patients. Among the studied neurotransmitters, increased serotonin and glutamate as well as decreased levels of gamma-aminobutyric acid N-Acetylaspartate and oxytocin appear to have the most empirical evidence.

The authors assess the relationship between autism spectrum disorder symptomatology, theory of mind, and other individual factor on children's responses through a study attempting to determine the factors that contribute to the complexity of the emotion of embarrassment.

The closing study addresses that with respect to dietary issues, awareness of the eating habits and feeding problems experienced by autism spectrum disorder children needs to be emphasized among parents and guardians.

Chapter 1 - There is a great deal of misinformation about children with autism spectrum disorders (ASD) and auditory processing disorders (APD). Many parents search for things to do to help their children when they suspect or are told by some professional that their child has some APD problem. Yet, professionals telling parents of these problems in children often do not truly understand what auditory processing disorders are and how ASD can affect test findings or responses on rating forms. Additionally, professionals often do not provide formal, standardized tests of auditory processing for children with ASD. Some parents are told by other professionals that their children with ASD cannot be assessed for APD leaving the parents lost regarding how to help their children who may have problems processing what they hear. This chapter discusses what auditory processing disorders are really all about, how APD problems can affect children with ASD, how children with ASD can be evaluated for the different types of APD, and, most importantly, what evidence-based treatments/therapies are appropriate to be used with children with ASD.

Chapter 2 - Hearing loss is the most common developmental abnormality present at birth in approximately two to four per 1000 newborns. The negative effects of undiagnosed hearing loss include delayed language, learning, and speech development. Approximately 40% of children with hearing loss will have an accompanying disorder according to a recent epidemiological report by Gallaudet Research Institute in 2009. Autism Spectrum Disorder (ASD) is a common neurodevelopmental disorder, which also negatively affects communication and social interaction. Interestingly, the prevalence of ASD in the general population is 1 in 68 but rises to 1 in 59 in children with hearing loss. The chapter will highlight the relationship between ASD and hearing loss and the challenges associated with making a dual diagnosis. It will discuss specific anatomical differences in the central auditory pathway and brain, the auditory processing of acoustic stimuli in children with ASD, and the audiological management of children with ASD, including hypersensitivity.

Chapter 3 - Developmental approaches characterized interventions based on the typical sequences of the child's development, paying particular attention to the linguistic, motor and socio-emotional aspects, within a relational perspective. The purpose of this paper was to identify developmental interventions for children with Autism Spectrum Disorders (ASD) aged between 0 and 12 years old. A literature review was carried out searching on MEDLINE, PsycINFO, and PsycARTICLES and manually on key journals and reference lists of key articles. All the electronic databases have been consulted by setting a range of year of publication between 2009 and 2019, and only articles in English have been considered. Two reviewers assessed studies against predetermined inclusion criteria and 72 unique studies met the authors' inclusion criteria. The interventions selected were described and the main outcomes discussed. This review highlights the need for improved research on intervention programs and the important service needs for families and children with Autism Spectrum Disorders.

Chapter 4 - Children with autism spectrum disorder (ASD) often have fewer opportunities to participate in play than typically developing children because of their tendencies for repetitive play behaviours and preference for independent play. The Holland Bloorview (HB) *FIRST*® robotics program embeds technology into a playful activity that was designed to be accessible for children with disabilities. The objectives of the study included: (1) to measure pediatric volition among children with ASD participating in the robotics program, and (2) an exploratory objective to observe volitional behaviours among children with ASD in the robotics program. This study used a mixed-method design with a pediatric volitional questionnaire, video recordings and structured observations of 6 consecutive workshops. The results showed that pediatric volition had no statistically significant change in the total median score from the beginning to the end of the robotics program. However, through the observations children showed patterns of demonstrating interest and enjoyment of participating in the program.

Chapter 5 - Autism spectrum condition (ASC) has been widely studied in literature, but many questions still need to be answered regarding how neurotransmitters are involved and how they are related to ASC psychopathology. A review was carried out in order to describe the main neurotransmitters in ASC patients. Among the studied neurotransmitters, increased serotonin and glutamate as well as decreased levels of gamma-aminobutyric acid N-Acetylaspartate and oxytocin appeared to have the most empirical evidence in ASC. Additional neurotransmitters as norepinephrine, acetylcholine, cortisol, and endogenous opioids have also been associated with ASC but there is still little support for the underlying mechanisms. Measurement of these neurotransmitters was usually obtained from different types of biological samples such as plasma, urine, or cerebrospinal fluid. Moreover, recent neuro-imaging techniques are also being used, providing a more precise and informative measure of neurotransmitter system functioning in ASC. Thus, several studies have described neurotransmitters' alterations in ASC patients. Overall, amino acid neurotransmitters, especially increased levels of serotonin, have shown more evidence for playing a role in ASC etiopathogenesis. Therefore, further neurotransmitter research is needed in order to elucidate the underlying mechanisms of ASC neuropathology, supporting a more comprehensive and theory-based approach of this disorder. Finally, measurement of these neurotransmitters and studies to search for new biomarkers may become a potential target for helping clinicians with early ASC diagnosis and treatment.

Chapter 6 - Factors that contribute to the complexity of the emotion of embarrassment were studied in this research. Twenty-three children with Autism Spectrum Disorders (ASD) and 25 neurotypical children were asked to complete an embarrassment measure that tapped into three faucets of their understanding of embarrassment. Specifically, the authors examined whether children were aware of the role of the audience when asked to imagine themselves in embarrassing situations, whether they were able to distinguish between intense and mildly embarrassing situations happening to another child, and the extent to which children could recount their own embarrassing experiences. Additionally, this study assessed the relations between ASD symptomatology, theory of mind (ToM), and other individual factors (FSIQ, age) on children's responses across the embarrassment tasks. When asked to imagine themselves in an embarrassing situation, all of the children labeled the active (derisive) audience vignette to be the most embarrassing and the vignette with no audience to be the least embarrassing. However, children with ASD were significantly more likely to find the passive audience (i.e., an audience is present but makes no comment) vignette to be embarrassing. Children with ASD were also less accurate in identifying and recounting embarrassing situations than neurotypical children. Greater ToM ability was correlated with a better understanding of embarrassment in children with ASD, especially when asked to imagine themselves in an embarrassing scenario with a derisive audience present. Greater ASD symptomatology was also correlated with a less accurate understanding of embarrassment in this same condition. The present study's implications and future research directions are discussed.

Chapter 7 - Autism Spectrum Disorder (ASD) is the fastest growing developmental disability that affects children particularly prior to the age of three in the areas of verbal & non-verbal communication, social interactions, physical abnormalities, sensory impairments & cognitive function. Along with these issues, dietary risk factors also affect the normal development of the children which make them vulnerable to serious nutritional deficiencies. Diet related issues like gastro-intestinal complications, leaky-guts; micro-biota composition, food neo-phobia, selective or picky eating habits and certain foods (gluten, casein) could aggravate with the symptoms of ASD and could be developed into a major and recurrent concern as reported by the parents or caretakers of ASD. Despite recent advances in the diagnostic tools & knowledge of pivotal factors, the exact etiology of autism remains unidentified, but it is predicted to be due to exposure to genetic susceptibility, medical co-morbidities & other environmental factors. Presently there is no known therapy to treat ASD, however children with this disorder do progress & the diverse symptoms related to it can be improved with primary intervention & treatments. Professionals researching on ASD have clearly indicated that early diagnosis & intervention programs including the pharmacological & non-conventional methods viz;

occupational, pragmatic skills along with dietary modifications may lead to significant improvement outcomes & better levels of functioning for children with ASD, as they reach their adulthood. Dietary related risk factors & how food plays a pivotal role in reducing the symptoms of ASD is the new emerging area of research work which has to be substantially validated through evidence based diets. With respect to dietary issues, awareness on eating habits and feeding problems experienced by ASD children need to be emphasized among parents or guardians of children as the road to recovery in every ailment is through diet.

In: Understanding Children with Autism … ISBN: 978-1-53617-647-6
Editor: Anne Bourque 

*Chapter 1*

# AUDITORY PROCESSING DISORDERS AND CHILDREN WITH AUTISM SPECTRUM DISORDER

***Jay R. Lucker****

Department of Communication Sciences and Disorders,
Howard University, Washington, DC, US

## ABSTRACT

There is a great deal of misinformation about children with autism spectrum disorders (ASD) and auditory processing disorders (APD). Many parents search for things to do to help their children when they suspect or are told by some professional that their child has some APD problem. Yet, professionals telling parents of these problems in children often do not truly understand what auditory processing disorders are and how ASD can affect test findings or responses on rating forms. Additionally, professionals often do not provide formal, standardized tests of auditory processing for children with ASD. Some parents are told by other professionals that their children with ASD cannot be assessed for APD

* Corresponding Author's E-mail: apddrj@verizon.net.

leaving the parents lost regarding how to help their children who may have problems processing what they hear.

This chapter discusses what auditory processing disorders are really all about, how APD problems can affect children with ASD, how children with ASD can be evaluated for the different types of APD, and, most importantly, what evidence-based treatments/therapies are appropriate to be used with children with ASD.

**Keywords:** auditory processing disorders, autism spectrum disorders, evaluation, treatment

## INTRODUCTION

Parents who have children with autism spectrum disorder (ASD), also just called autism, often observe that their children are not listening or are not able to understand what is said to them. Many times, these children are observed covering their ears when they hear certain sounds, such as loud, unexpected noises. Other times they may see their children losing control and having negative emotional and behavioral reactions when such noises are present. When the parents ask their medical doctors, psychologists, teachers or other professionals who work with their child about the parents' concerns, these professionals say that this is typical of a child with ASD, and they recommend using ear plugs, earphones/headphones, and removing the child from the environment in which the noise is present.

Trying to get a better understanding of what is going on with children with ASD, parents, and professionals, may search the internet for information regarding listening problems and what may be helpful for the child with ASD. They may come across websites from autism organizations in which they make statements that children with ASD have deficits in auditory processing which can interfere with the child learning to tolerate sounds which may not even be loud or annoying to the parents or other children who do not have ASD. For example, *Autism Speaks* is funding research looking at auditory processing disorders in children with ASD. Their website discussing auditory processing and ASD states the following (https://www.autismspeaks.org/expert-opinion/autism-and-auditory-processing-disorder-whats-connection):

> If you have autism – or have a child with autism – you may have experienced or seen indications of this difficulty such as the following:
>
> - Covering one's ears in situations that don't seem particularly noisy to most people
> - Humming in response to chatter or other noises
> - Feeling distressed when surrounded by a lot of chatter or other noise
>
> Parents often notice these "auditory hypersensitivities" when their children are quite young – even before a child is diagnosed with autism.

This website also provides a typical description of auditory processing (also called central auditory processing) and cites one of the professional associations that is involved with auditory processing and its disorders, the American Speech-Language-Hearing Association (ASHA). In that description, they present a picture of the typical central auditory pathway from the ear to the auditory center of the cortex in the brain. What is shown is how the neural information is transmitted from the ear, through the lower brainstem, then, through the higher brainstem (thalamus) projecting to the auditory cortex. However, as the reader with see later in this chapter, there is more to auditory processing than merely this central auditory pathway, and research supports that children with ASD may have problems processing what they hear due to what is known as problems with the nonclassical auditory pathway which does not transmit neural information from the upper brainstem to the auditory cortex, but transmits that information to a very different part of the brain which leads to the negative emotional and behavioral reactions parents may see with their children with ASD.

If parents read websites or other publications that identify that children with ASD have auditory processing disorders (APD) they may choose to agree with the professionals who recommend plugging up the child's ears to avoid having the child hear the sounds that contribute to negative emotional and behavioral reactions as well as avoid exposing their child with ASD to environments in which such sounds may be present. However, loud and annoying sounds can suddenly "pop-up" without expectation in many environments. For example, merely walking down the street with their child, the parents may notice their child's negative reactions when, suddenly, a siren from a fire engine or police car is heard in the distance. Even going to a quiet park to allow their child to play, there may suddenly come a group of children verbally reacting to their excitement being at the park making very happy, loud sounds which lead to their child with ASD to react negatively. What parents may consider is to seek a professional, such as an occupational therapist (OT), who suggests that one treatment for children with ASD which improves the child's overall functioning is the use of a listening therapy. These listening therapies can help reduce some of the negative emotional and, thus, behavioral reactions to sounds, but the parents may be led to believe that the completion of the listening therapy will contribute to general improvements in the child's overall behavior and even increase the child's verbal skills and understanding of what is said to the child. However, these professionals often do not provide evidence-based research to support the general improvements in the children's behavior, communication, and listening skills after completing such listening therapies. There is research that supports the use of listening therapies to reduce negative emotional reactions to sounds which opens the auditory system to be more willing to take in and process what the child hears. Then, other behavioral therapy to reduce negative behavioral reactions and increase listening comprehension and verbal communication can be successfully provided to the child. This chapter discusses evidence-based research supporting the concept that the auditory processing hypersensitivity problems seen with children having ASD is not an auditory based but an emotional based issue, and that listening therapies may reduce the negative emotional reactions so that behavioral therapies can successfully change the child's reactions when hearing these loud and annoying sounds. But, first, let's take a look at what goes on when we process auditory information including the multiple systems involved, one being the emotional system.

## How Does the Brain Process What It Hears?

The standard approach to auditory processing (see Figure 1) is related to what was discussed above that may be presented on websites about children with ASD. Professional associations, such as the American Speech-Language-Hearing Association (ASHA) (2005) and the American Academy of Audiology (AAA) (2010), have published papers describing their understanding and approach to auditory processing and its disorders. The approach these associations accept is as follows. Auditory information is first picked up by the right and left ears so long as hearing is normal. The information is converted to neural impulses in the inner ear, called the cochlea, and then transmitted from the cochlea to the low brainstem auditory level via the auditory nerve ($8^{th}$ cranial nerve). The low brainstem starts some of the early processing of that neural information and transmits this processed neural information to higher brainstem regions until the information reaches the upper brainstem, the thalamic level. From this thalamic region, after additional processing occurs, the neural information is transmitted to the right and left auditory cortices in the brain. The two cortices connect with each other via white neural fibers called the corpus callosum. It is at this level that auditory processing ends according to these professional associations. The higher levels of processing (discussed next) are said to not be related to auditory processing specifically but involve other factors. Thus, understanding this approach, the concept would be that children with ASD who are overly sensitive to sounds have a problem somewhere in processing at either the low brainstem, upper brainstem, thalamic, cortical, or interhemispheric corpus callosum levels. But, none of these levels involves emotional and behavioral reactions. Thus, the question arises whether there is more involved in auditory processing than merely this central auditory pathway.

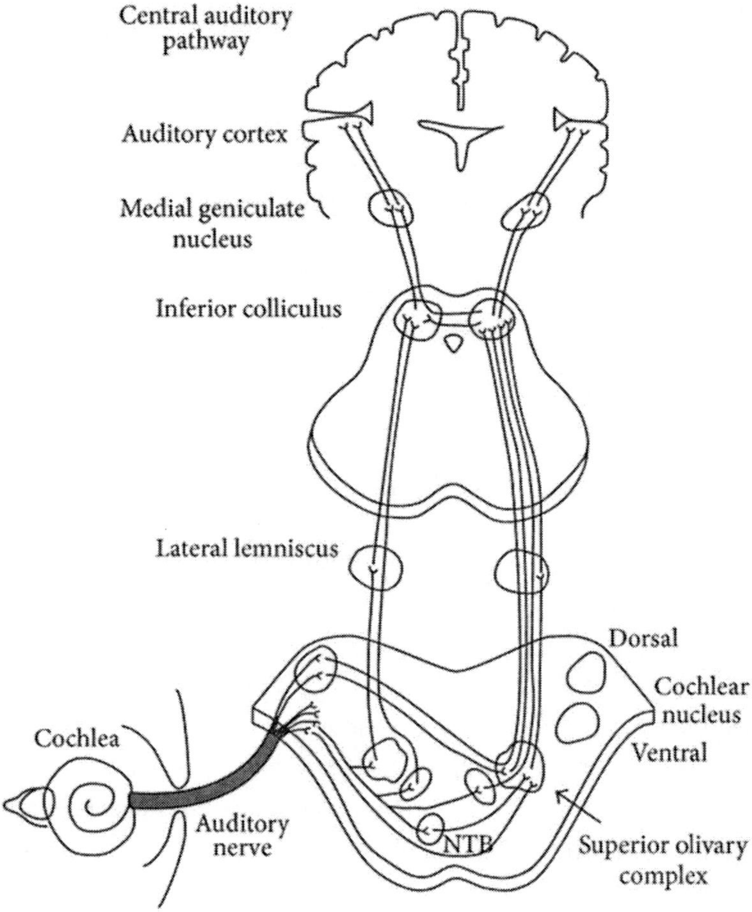


Figure 1. Classic Central Auditory Pathway. (Creative Commons Attribution 3.0 Unported) From Lucker Doman 2015, 2.

Many years ago, in 1977, at the first National Conference on Auditory Processing Disorders in Cincinnati, OH (Auditory Processing Disorder 1977) and in the early 1980s, at the Einstein Medical Center in the Bronx, NY, the author presented his initial understanding of auditory processing and its disorders. This approach differs from the AAA and ASHA approaches in the following way. These professional organizations view auditory processing involving only one system, the central auditory nervous system. In contrast, the Lucker MultiSystem Integrative Approach (LMSIA)

(Edell, Lucker, Alderman 2009 (Chapter 2); Hawkins and Lucker 2018 (5-9)) views auditory processing involving multiple systems as follows.

The LMSIA description begins with the ear, the eighth nerve and the central auditory pathway but includes other systems of the brain. While the incoming auditory information is processed through the brainstem up to the auditory cortices, there is also processing occurring in other systems. For example, having visual information regarding what a person may be discussing in that person's verbal message, the listener uses the visual input to aid in comprehending what the person is saying. For example, if the speaker is describing a car, and there is only one car in the area in which the speaker and listener are communicating, much of what the speaker says will relate to that car. If the listener is looking at the car while the speaker is presenting the description, the listener will have a much easier time relating what the speaker is saying to the information being presented. Additionally, knowing the topic of the discussion, the cognitive and linguistic systems of the brain start to highlight factors that may be associated with the person's verbal input and modify these cognitive and linguistic factors based on the auditory information being processed. There is also a level of attention involving frontal lobe executive functioning so the listener is attending appropriately to what the person is saying and is sending neural impulses down to lower brainstem levels of the central auditory pathways to get filters to work to screen out or block the unimportant/distracting sounds from being processed to higher levels so that what is processed at higher levels is the important, relevant information. Additionally, since auditory information is sensory information, the sensory gating systems of the brain are involved in ensuring that appropriate auditory information is processed higher while irrelevant auditory information is filtered out.

The last system discussed is our emotional system in the limbic system of the brain that is not part of the traditional central auditory pathways. It is the pathway from the upper brainstem to the emotional system that has been identified as the nonclassical auditory pathway (see Figure 2). In Lucker's LMSIA approach (, Lucker 2017 (4-12) & 2018 (5-9)), and related to children with ASD, this nonclassical pathway is very important regarding what likely is going on with children with ASD when they react to sounds, especially sounds to which they have negative emotional reactions.

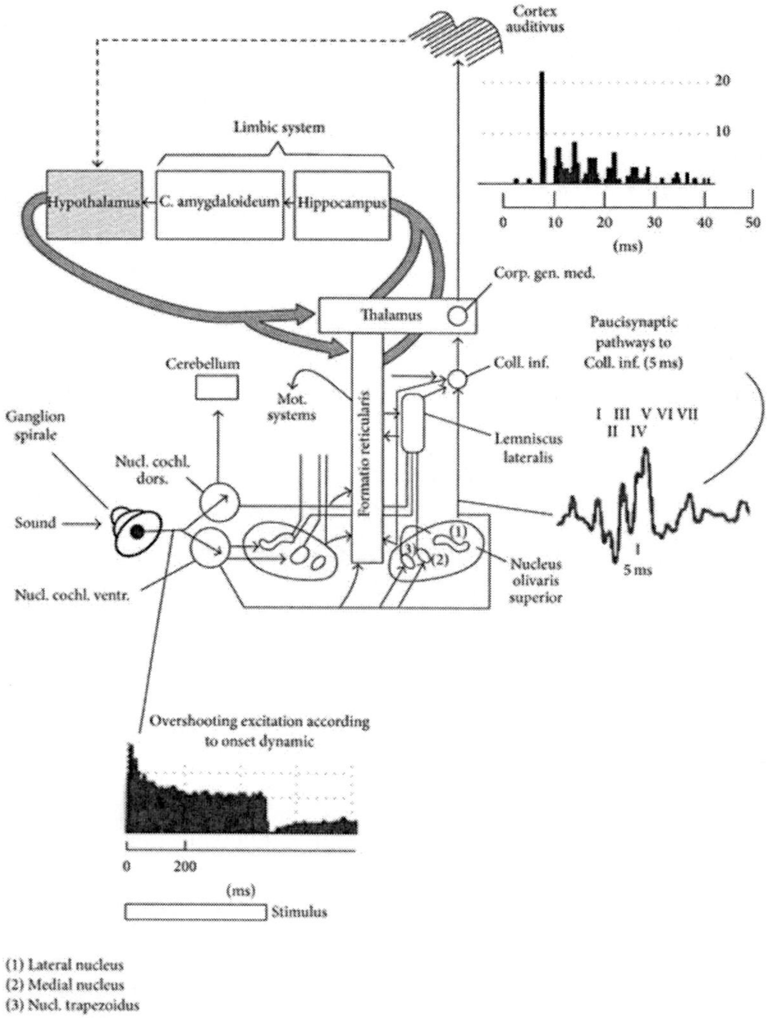


Figure 2. Nonclassical central auditory pathway (Creative Commons Attribution 3.0 Unported) From Lucker Doman 2015, 3.

Moller and associates (2002 (41-44) & 2005 (625-629) identified that from the upper brainstem central auditory pathway, not only are there connections to higher cortical levels, but the nonclassical auditory pathway connects the central auditory pathway at this upper brainstem level with the emotional centers of the brain in what is known as the limbic system. Thus, before higher level auditory, cognitive, linguistic, memory, and other systems are involved in processing what we hear, the emotional system receives the auditory input and starts to process that information. Additionally, connections from the auditory cortices on both sides of the brain connect with this emotional system. Thus, when we hear sounds, we may have emotional reactions to those sounds. A great example is music. Most of us would agree that there is music that is very emotionally relaxing, while other music is emotionally irritating and can be scary. Imagine a child with ASD hearing sounds that are confusing or annoying to the young child. These sounds can set off negative emotional reactions. Sounds, such as loud sounds, and sudden unexpected sounds can set off strong negative emotional reactions from the limbic system in the child's brain.

In addition to this emotional reacting system, there is a mechanism for emotional memory. Thus, imagine that the child hears a sound that leads to negative emotional reactions. The emotional memory center of the child's limbic system (known as the amygdala) may hold on to the memory of this negative "sound" and generalize the negativity to similar sounds and, later, to many other sounds. The emotional memory system may decide that many sounds could lead to negative emotional reactions, and the child's autonomic nervous system responds negatively often with what is called the "fight or flight response." This response could contribute to the child being fearful of all sounds, most sounds, sounds of a specific loudness level (such as all sounds louder than a normal conversational speaking level) or sounds that are unpredictable when they occur (like the siren of the fire engine or police car or the banging of the door as it closes). Since many typical environmental sounds can fall into the categories of "fearful sounds," the child with ASD may have negative emotional reactions to many different sounds. If the annoying fearful sounds occur in specific environments, the child could become fearful of those environments even if there were no sounds in these environments. These over reactions are often referred to as over sensitivity and, when it comes to sounds and listening, we call it hypersensitivity or hypersensitive hearing. Some have called these hypersensitivities phonophobia which would translate to fear (phobia) of sound (phono).

## How auditory Hypersensitivity Can Be Assessed in Children with ASD

Auditory hypersensitivity is often evaluated by professionals merely by asking parents, teachers, and others who interact with children who have ASD about their observations of the children. Yet, these observations and reports are subjective. That is, they involve the reporter to identify what they interpret based on the child's behaviors seen when the child reacts in certain ways, typically negatively. Yet there are formal, standardized behavioral tests that can be completed to determine whether a child may have auditory hypersensitivity. Audiologists use these measures when they fit hearing aids; but rarely do they use them just to assess a person's listening and sensitivity to sound.

The typical methods audiologists use to assess sensitivity to sound, especially loud sounds, is through measures called Uncomfortable Listening Level (UCL), Loudness Discomfort Level (LDL) or just loudness tolerance. The author published a research study looking at UCL/LDL measures in children with ASD. The author presented the standard audiological tolerance testing as follows. Using noises (called narrow band noises) and tones that warble (such as the sound of some sirens) which have specific frequencies (related to pitch in our perception of the sounds), he varied the intensity (loudness) of the sounds. The sounds started at what would be a loudness level around loud conversational speaking (70dBHL) and increased to the maximal loudness of the audiological equipment (called the audiometer) which was between 100 and 110dBHL depending on the frequency used. To better understand these loudness levels, consider the following. The Occupational Safety and Health Administration (OSHA) (n.d.) has tables relating sounds (based on a scale called the dBA). The dBA scale relates to how sound is heard by the human ear. It is approximately 10dB louder than the dBHL scale which relates our hearing of sound for specific frequencies rather than the overall sound that things make (which is what the dBA scale measures). For example, 100dBHL would be approximately 110dBA while 110dBHL would be approximately 120dBA. Thus, a 100dBHL sound would be about as loud as night club with music or a music concert); 110dBHL would be about as loud as a person operating heavy equipment would hear if the person were not wearing earmuffs.

Based on the loudness tolerance tested by the author (Lucker 2013), about two-thirds of children diagnosed with ASD had no problems tolerating 110dBHL of sound at each of the frequencies tested for both the noises and tones used when the children were engaged in the listening task. However, the question arises how would the author identify if the child could not tolerate the sounds? The one-third of children with ASD who were identified as not tolerating the loud sounds were observed to react negatively in facial expression, body language, or even pulling the earphones off their heads while the other children continued to engage in the "game" that was used to evaluate if the child heard and responded to the sounds. Since all the children with ASD were able to play the game appropriately so that their hearing thresholds could be measured, the children were engaged appropriately in the same game, but the sounds differed from the hearing threshold testing that used very soft sounds. The author concluded that most children with ASD do not have problems dealing auditorily with loud sounds; their negative emotional reactions were more their emotional systems' responses to the sounds in the environments in which the sounds are heard. Also, the children were positively engaged in the "game" used to evaluate their hearing which was also the "game" used to evaluate their tolerance of loud sounds. The conclusion the author drew was that auditory hypersensitivity is more an emotional reaction than an auditory or hearing based reaction. Later in this chapter, the author discusses children who do not respond to sound at all (called auditory hyposensitivity) and what this indicates and how it may involve auditory processing in these children. Thus, the focus of treatment is to reduce the negative emotional reaction in these children.

## WAYS PEOPLE MAY DEAL WITH AUDITORY HYPERSENSITIVITY IN CHILDREN WITH ASD

As stated earlier, the usual way people deal with children with ASD who show sound sensitivities is to have the child avoid the sounds. Professionals often recommend such avoidance to parents of children with ASD. The avoidance recommendations include actual avoidance, such as not bring the child to a shopping mall or avoid going to the playground when others are in the playground, or not going to the playground at all. Since it is sometimes difficult to avoid such situations, or it is desirable to allow the child to be in such places (such as the playground or at school), the recommendation made is to have the child wear ear plugs or headphones that block out sound in such environments. What is interesting to consider is what do such recommendations teach the child, and how may the child's system interpret the use of such avoidance techniques.

To best understand what can occur, consider the following. Imagine you have a child who is afraid of flying in an airplane. What you could do is avoid having the child fly in airplanes? Over time the child may become fearful of going to the airport because the child may think that the parent will make the child get on an airplane and fly away. So, the family avoids going to the airport with the child. But the fear of flying and, now, airports, becomes generalized to a fear of even being near an airport. So, the family avoids going near airports with the child even if it means finding other ways to drive from point A to point B if the normal drive would pass an airport that can be visualized from the car. Over time, the child may also become fearful when airplanes are flying in the sky. Would the family then avoid having the child go out of the house since the family lives close to an airport and planes are flying overhead every day? Or would the family move from their home to another location far from any airport or from planes flying overhead? We can go on with this discussion, but the focus is that what started as a fear of flying in an airplane became a greater fear to the degree of even a fear of leaving the house or having to move to another location.

The avoidance response does not help the child overcome the fear of flying. What many psychologists recommend is a method called systematic desensitization (Dubord 2011; Head and Gross 2009) in which the child is systematically introduced to negative factors until the child's system overcomes the fear to a degree that either the child is no longer frightened or is more willing to deal with the factor being avoided. The outcome of systematic desensitization behavioral therapy is that the child no longer has negative emotional reactions to the stimuli that caused the fear or the child's system has learned to deal successfully with the fear. As the name, systematic desensitization, indicates, the training is done systematically in steps to desensitize the system to the negative emotional reactions that occurred. Many children who have undergone systematic desensitization find they no longer are fearful of the stimuli which they previously feared, or they can deal successfully with such stimuli. Additionally, their acceptance of things they previously avoided and feared often generalizes to many other situations expanding their acceptance of situations they previously avoided.

Research using systematic desensitization has been used on children with ASD (Koegel Openden Koegel 2004; Lucker 2013; Lucker Doman 2012; Stiegler Davis 2010). The research has shown that children with ASD who were fearful of specific sounds could be desensitized and start to accept hearing those sounds. Additionally, their fears of other sounds start to reduce even if the behavioral therapy does not specifically focus on those sounds. This latter factor is called generalization. What appears to occur is that the emotional system of the brain starts to re-learn that the sounds to which the child was fearful are no longer frightening. The training often focuses on giving the child another appropriate behavior to use when the sound is present and to control the child's behavior so that their emotional systems learn that they can control their reactions/behaviors, and the emotional memory system learns to remember that they were not "hurt." Through such training, the child's emotional system learns that the sounds are no longer fearful, and they are no longer overly sensitive to such sounds and the environments in which the sounds occur.

To better understand how systematic desensitization can reduce negative emotional reactions, the following example is provided. The author was asked to consult on a case of a young boy diagnosed with ASD who was enrolled in a special education program at a school. The parent and teachers were very concerned with the child's strong avoidance and "flight" responses when loud and annoying sounds were present in the classroom. One such sound was the fire alarm that was used in the school. One concern identified by the teacher was that at the beginning of the school year, the school had fire drills to practice what students should do if the fire alarm were to go off. The first fire drill occurred and the boy had strong negative emotional reactions which required one of the teaching assistants to wait in the classroom to monitor the child to ensure that he did no damage to things or hurt himself after he started negatively reacting to the fire alarm. Fortunately, the aide worked well to keep the boy safe.

During a conference with the parent and teachers, this professional suggested that what could be done is to engage the child with the alarm sound (that is, give him control of the sound and desensitize him to the loud, annoying fire alarm). From this conversation, it was identified that the child loved numbers. Thus, the author suggested to have the child count the number of times the alarm rang. Thus, if the alarm went off "gong-gong-gong," the boy would say it rang three times. One of the aides worked with the boy during the school day to practice counting sounds. Starting with the aide saying sounds like "bong-bong-bong" and then moving to actual sounds such as tapping or hitting the table, or the sound of a buzz from the cell phone and moving on to the sound of a bell. Each time hearing the sound the boy counted the number of times the sound was heard. He was rewarded initially for just counting the sounds and, overtime, for reporting the total number of sounds he heard.

The teacher was informed (after a few weeks in which the behavioral counting training was practiced) that there would be a fire alarm at a specific time that day. Ten minutes before the fire alarm, the boy was told that there was going to be a buzz sound, and the teacher needed to know how many times the buzz sounded. Five minutes before the fire alarm, the child was told, again, to remember to count the buzz and report to the teacher how many times the bell rang. The class, as a whole, also practiced lining up and walking outside to where they were to wait when the fire alarm went off.

The time came and the fire alarm started buzzing. The teaching assistant reminded the child to count the buzzes and report to her how many times the bell rang while he was to line up and walk with the class outside. During this line up and walking, the teaching aid noticed the child counting. The boy cooperated with the class, lined up appropriately, marched outside, and continued his counting. When the alarm stopped, the boy leaned over to his teacher and said a number. The teacher looked questionably at the boy and told him to be quiet, but the teaching assistant, overhearing the boy saying the number, responded to the boy, "Good job" and gave him a high five (to indicate great work) and then reinforced he had to be quiet. The teacher asked the children to take their seats, but the boy would not leave the teacher's side. The teacher turned to the boy and asked why he was standing there. He responded repeating the number. The teacher then remembered that the boy was to tell her how many times the alarm rang. She then praised the boy for counting. Thus, the desensitization gave the boy something he enjoyed (positive feedback) which was counting things, and he did his duty by counting the buzzes during the fire drill. What this example shows is how a child with ASD can go from strong negative emotional (flight) reactions to being engaged and involved appropriately in a task even when a loud, annoying sound was heard. Thus, teaching a child how to control behavior and engage in the listening task can desensitize the child, and the practice (systematically) can teach the child behaviors that are appropriate when such loud and annoying sounds are heard.

## USE OF LISTENING THERAPIES

For many children with ASD, either prior to or along with the systematic desensitization they need to first open their auditory systems because their "systems" have closed down because of the fear of sounds that may be heard. What some professionals recommend is that children with auditory sound sensitivities start their treatments with what is called a listening therapy.

These therapies can include (alphabetically) Integrated Listening Systems (iLS) (www.integratedlistening.com), The Listening Program (TLP) (www.advancedbrain.com), Therapeutic Listening also known as Vital Links (www.vitallinks.net), Tomatis Therapy (www.tomatis.com), and some others. Research exists on these specific listening therapies demonstrating significant improvements in auditory processing abilities in children who have completed each of these listening training programs (Chakraborty Kaf Lucker, 2018, 1-9; Lucker Doman 2012, 103-108; Lucker Doman 2013, 184-191; Lucker Doman 2015, 1-8; Lucker Doman 2019, 48-54; Reeves and Lucker 2017,6-9; Vargas and Lucker 2016). For example, the author has investigated two of these programs (iLS and TLP) finding very significant improvements in auditory processing for children who completed the programs. In many of these publications, the authors discuss how a listening therapy can reduce hypersensitivity in children. In some publications, the authors also discuss the use of a listening therapy and systematic desensitization improving listening abilities and reducing hypersensitivity and negative emotional reactions in children with ASD.

In a publication by coauthors Lucker and Doman (2015, 1-8), the specific systems involved in auditory hypersensitivity are described. Most of the systems involve the limbic system and the autonomic nervous system (ANS). One of the main systems involved is called the vagus nerve. Porges (2011) presented what he calls the Polyvagal Theory involving this cranial nerve showing the many areas innervated by this nerve. When we consider that when we have negative emotional reactions, we have difficulties speaking, problems breathing, feeling upset in our stomach's etc., it is interesting to see that the vagus nerve innervates each of these areas of our body.

Using his Polyvagal Theory, Porges developed a listening program he calls the Safe and Sound Protocol (SSP) (https://integrated listening.com/ssp-safe-sound-protocol-clinical-resources/). Although distributed by the company that produces iLS, the SSP program differs from iLS in the number of days in which the therapy is to be done as well as what music is used and how the music was recorded. The iLS program can involve months of therapy while SSP is completed over five days for one hour of listening per day. Thus, for children who have strong, negative emotional reactions to sounds and listening, one might try SSP. However, other listening therapies cited above can be used but must be completed for many months.

What the author is presenting here is that children with ASD who have auditory hypersensitivity typically show negative emotional reactions to sound. What the research on listening therapies indicates is that these negative emotional reactions can be reduced, and the listening system opened after completing a listening therapy. Then, desensitization can be provided giving the child's system control over the listening situation so that the child no longer has these strong negative emotional reactions when sounds that were annoying prior to these treatments are heard.

## Auditory Hyposensitivity

Not all children with ASD show auditory hypersensitivity. Many children with ASD do not respond to sound unless (a) they are prompted to do so and (b) they have been trained to respond in a specific way when specific sound stimuli are present. Other children with ASD do not at all respond when they hear sound or when people speak with them. These children can be identified having auditory hyposensitivity. "Hypo" means under or "no" so that hyposensitivity indicates that these children are not responsive to sound.

During audiological testing, what is typically done is to try to get children to respond to the presence of sound they hear. For children with hyposensitive hearing, they do not learn to respond to the sounds and would need many special behavioral training sessions to learn to respond to the specific sounds used in audiological hearing testing. However, since audiological tests measure different frequencies or pitches of sound, the children would need to be trained to respond to each frequency that will be used in the hearing testing. Thus, these children often are identified as having hearing loss or being "deaf" when attempts are made to do standard hearing (audiological) tests. However, when objective electrophysiological measures of hearing are used that do not require a child's reactions, hearing is found to be normal.

What is hypothesized with these children with ASD who show no reactions to sounds is that their early emotional responses to sounds become generalized to be negative to all sounds since sound, especially during infancy, is a bombardment of auditory stimuli which their brains may not be able to tolerate. Thus, sound, in general, may be interpreted as negative leading to the emotional system memory in the limbic system to interpret all, or most, sound as being intolerable. Thus, the emotional system sends neural impulses to the brainstem auditory system not to process sound so that sound, even loud sounds, are ignored by the brain. This could explain why children with ASD who are hyposensitive do not learn to respond to sound the way typically developing kids' brains learn to respond to sound. These children also are not well able to be trained to respond to sound even when carefully controlled behavioral training is employed.

For children with auditory hyposensitivity we still need to reduce the negative emotional interpretation of sound and remove the "shut-down" reaction from emotional memory. These children may also benefit from a listening therapy such as the one's discussed earlier. These children would then be ready to learn to respond to sound and learn to put meaning to sound even if they can only learn the meaning using behavioral treatments. However, these children may also learn to generalize the responses they learn to sound to use in similar situations, called generalizing.

## Auditory Processing in Chidlren with ASD Who Do Not Have Hyper- or Hypo- Sensitivity

There are many children with ASD who do respond appropriately to sound and are not overly (hyper-) sensitive or under (hypo-) sensitive. These children learn to put meaning to sound and learn to respond to auditory stimuli. However, many of these children may still have problems appropriately processing what they hear. They would not show the indications of auditory hyper- or hypo- sensitivity discussed above, but they would have problems in other areas of auditory processing. For these children, they can complete a comprehensive auditory processing assessment which primarily involves that they identify through picture pointing or repeating what they hear that they can process auditory stimuli. Some auditory processing tests require some degree of manipulation of what is heard which children with higher functioning ASD can complete while other children with ASD cannot complete. The following are some of the more common areas of auditory processing found to be deficient among children with moderate to high functioning ASD.

## Auditory Extraction and Overloading

One area of auditory processing often found to be deficient in these higher functioning children with ASD is auditory extraction. Extraction involves the brain's abilities to pull out the key auditory information in messages that carry the meaning of the whole message. There are three different types of extraction. The first type is the most common one found among children with ASD by the author. This type is called auditory temporal extraction. Temporal relates to time and time involves "rhythm" or tempo (thus, temporal). For example, when we speak, we may say a number of things quickly. Consider realizing you are late for something and telling your child you are going out, so you want the child to put on the child's jacket and get some item the child often carries. Because you are late, you might speak quickly. The child goes to get the jacket, but that is all the child does, and a few minutes later you go to the child and see that your child is still looking in the closet but seems lost. Your verbal message came too quickly for the child's brain to process it all, remember and formulate appropriate responses to what you have said, and complete the direction provided. There are specific auditory processing tests that look at auditory temporal processing as well as therapy specific to this disorder.

Another problem for children with auditory temporal processing is the ability to understand how the rhythm of what people say changes the emotional meaning of the message. For example, consider the message you might have said discussed above. If you are merely going outside, you might speak slower but also your rhythm would be more in the form of a direction or instruction. In contrast, because you are late and rushing to get out, not only are you speaking quickly, but the rhythm of what you say could be misinterpreted by a child with ASD who has temporal processing problems as indicating you are upset with the child or "yelling" at the child. This rhythm differentiates statements from demands and from humor and sarcasm. Thus, identifying whether a child with ASD has auditory temporal extraction problems is very important so that treatment for the speed of processing of auditory information can be provided along with language therapy focusing on teaching the child how to differentiate statements such as pure statements from statements indicating specific emotional factors and from humor and sarcasm. One such treatment is called Interactive Metronome or IM training (www.interactivemetronome.com). The author has engaged in research projects on IM training which have all shown that children completing such training significantly improve in their speed of processing of auditory information as well as improve in their comprehension of what is said to them (Chakborty, Kaf, and Lucker 2018, 1-9; Reeves and Lucker 2017, 6-9).

Another type of auditory extraction problem found with many children with ASD is called auditory lexical extraction. Lexical relates to words, so lexical extraction involves hearing and processing the key, important words in verbal messages. For example, consider you tell your child to get his jacket and meet you at the front door. The key words might be, "get jacket" – "meet at front door" – "hurry." Thus, the child does not have to remember and focus on every single word you say but only these seven key words even if the sentence you spoke was, "We are going out and need to hurry, so go get your jacket and meet me at the front door so we can go out." For children with ASD who can not do appropriate lexical (key word) extraction they only get part of the message and only put that part of the message into their memory. They become overloaded and overwhelmed and may have negative emotional reactions shutting down and just stand there doing nothing. There is also evaluation material that some audiologists may use to interpret auditory lexical extraction (also called decoding). Additionally, there are treatments for the overloading and teaching the child how to process the key words.

## Speech Understanding in Noise (SIN)

Another area of auditory processing most audiologists evaluate with children looks at the child's abilities to understand speech in the presence of noise (SIN). Even if the child with ASD does not have auditory hypersensitivity, the child may not have the neural processing abilities to pull out the relevant verbal message when noise is present. The noise becomes distracting, and the child loses the message.

One problem the author has seen in diagnosing SIN problems in children is that many audiologists only administer one test of SIN. If the child passes this one test, could it be possible that the child might fail other measures of SIN, and vice versa. Often what occurs is the test of SIN is done for each individual ear and the child passes for one ear and fails for the other ear, and the audiologist concludes that the child has problems filtering out the unwanted, distracting noise. But that is not an appropriate conclusion since the child passed for one of the two ears. This ear difference factor is discussed further below.

What the author recommends is that it is necessary to provide multiple measures of every aspect of auditory processing evaluated and to determine that this specific factor is not a problem by seeing if the child passes two out of three measures or is a problem because the child fails at least two out of three measures. Thus, in the above example, one measure of SIN found one ear normal and one ear failing so let's see what a second test indicates. Imagine the second test shows one ear is normal and one ear fails. The problem is more with the factor integrating the two ears and not due to filtering out the distracting noise. Or if the child fails one measure but passes two others, there are no problems with appropriate filtering, but the audiologist should see what factor accounted for the failure on the one test. Imagine the two measures passed uses single, monosyllabic words while the measure failed used sentences. The author would want to know if the child can appropriately repeat similar sentences without any noise present since the problem could be the amount of verbal information to be processed in the sentence (overloading or lexical extraction). Again, the main focus is that there are treatments for children who truly have SIN problems, so we want to appropriately identify if the child has a SIN problem. These treatments include practice identifying what a child hears when there is noise present with the noise increasing in volume and moving from general noise to linguistically meaningful distraction such as someone reading a story.

## Auditory Integrative Processing

The last area discussed in this chapter involves putting the pieces of auditory information together to form the meaningful whole which involves integrative processing. Auditory integration involves different systems in the brain working together harmoniously. Some of the measures of auditory integration are referred to as dichotic listening tasks. They usually use verbal material (numbers or words) presented to both ears with different numbers or words presented simultaneously to each ear evaluating auditory lexical (word) integration. Integrative processing is also evaluated by a few audiologists looking at how well a child is able to hear the individual phonemes (speech sounds) in words and put the sounds together to form the whole word (called auditory phonological integration). This process is important in reading decoding and spelling. Another aspect of phonological integration is hearing a whole word and identifying individual sounds in the words. This process is also important in reading and spelling. For example, consider what is involved when we learn rhyming words; we learn to drop the initial sound (so we need to identify the first or initial sound) and add a different sound to form the new word (involving blending the new sound into the word).

As stated above, problems with auditory phonological integration can affect reading and spelling abilities as well as children understanding what they hear when they hear new and unfamiliar words. Auditory lexical integration problems can affect comprehension of messages and memory since we remember the key pieces of information (extraction) and, later, put the pieces together to form the meaning of the whole message. There are treatments for both phonological integration and lexical integration. Additionally, if the dichotic functioning is found to be deficient, there is specific treatment for dichotic listening. Examples of programs that work on dichotic listening include the dichotic training part of the Acoustic Pioneer program (www.acousticpinoneer.com) and the CAPDOTS program (www.capdots.com). For phonological and lexical integration, there are programs such as Fast ForWord (www.scilearn.com). However, for both phonological and lexical integration problems, it is best to work with a professional, such as a speech-language pathologist or audiologist who provides specific training for auditory integrative processing deficits in children, especially those with ASD.

## Conclusion

There is a lot of information presented in this chapter because there are many different components of auditory processing, and the author wants the reader to understand these different components and how they can affect children with ASD. What is important for the reader to remember is the "S" in ASD means Spectrum. That is, there is no one thing as autism, but a spectrum of disorders. Some children with ASD are unsensitive to sound (hyposensitivity) while others may be overly sensitive (hypersensitivity) and treatment for each differs. Some are at a higher level of ASD so that they can take in and process auditory stimuli, but they do not know how to appropriately extract the words, or they get overloaded and overwhelmed with too much information or they cannot remember what they heard. Others cannot filter out unwanted noise so that they focus on the noise and cannot get the relevant verbal messages they hear or they cannot extract enough of the relevant message to place that information into memory and, later, integrate the pieces from memory to comprehend the meaning of the whole. Some children with ASD may have problems with reading and spelling because they have phonological integration problems. For some, information comes too quickly so they only get part of the message and, again, cannot comprehend the whole. For others, their temporal processing problems lead to their inability to understand the emotional factors in messages and to understand statements from questions, sarcasm, etc.

What the author hopes is that reading this chapter will help you better understand problems children with ASD may have relative to auditory processing abilities. Children with ASD may be observed having auditory processing problems, but the important factor is to identify what specific type of processing problems exist, how these can affect the child, and that there are accommodations and treatments that can be provided to help the child who has the specific type of auditory processing deficits described in this chapter. It is also hoped that the reader realizes that appropriate testing by qualified professionals is needed to identify the specific auditory processing deficits present so that appropriate treatments and accommodations can be provided.

This chapter focused mostly on what specific types of auditory processing may be found in children with ASD. How these types are identified and examples of some different treatments for children with different types of APD problems. However, identifying what treatments are needed for specific children with ASD requires a well trained and knowledgeable professional doing the auditory processing assessment who also understands ASD and relating specific treatments for specific types of APD problems. Thus, the reader is recommended to contact a professional who truly understands auditory processing and how it is to be assessed in children with ASD to find out how to obtain an appropriate assessment of a child with ASD and identify what specific interventions are needed for that child. Additionally, the reader may wish to read more about the author's approach and understanding of auditory processing disorders as they relate specifically to children with ASD (and Lucker 2018, 5-9; Lucker 2013, 2014a, b, c & d; 2018a & b; Lucker and Doman 2012).

## References


American Academy of Audiology 2010. *Clinical Practice Guidelines Diagnosis, Treatment and Management of Children and Adults with Central Auditory Processing Disorder*. Available from https://audiology-web.s3.amazonaws.com/migrated/CAPD%20Guidelines%208-2010.pdf_539952af956c79.73897613.pdf.

American Speech-Language-Hearing Association 2005. *Central Auditory Processing Disorders [Technical Report]*. Available from www.asha.org/policy.

Auditory Processing Disorder 1977. *History*. Accessed November 30, 2019. https://www.wikiwand.com/en/Auditory_processing_disorder#/History.

Chakraborty Sapna, Kaf, Wafaa, and Lucker Jay R. 2018. Interactive Metronome: Research review related to treating auditory processing disorders in children. *Journal of the Academy of Rehabilitative Audiology, XLX*, 1-9.

Dubord, Gregg 2011. Systematic desensitization. *Canadian Family Physician, 57*(11), 1299.

Edell, H, Lucker, JR, Alderman, L, (2009). *Don't You Get It? Living with Auditory Learning Disabilities* (Revised). Wood Dale, IL: Stoelting Company Publishers.

Hawkins, Jarin and Lucker, Jay R, 2018. Auditory processing disorders: A unifying definition and professional implications. *Topics in Central Auditory Processing, 3*(1), 5-9.

Head, Lara S, Gross, Alan Michael 2009. Systematic desensitization. In WT O'Donohue and JE Fisher (Eds.) *General Principles and Empirically Supported Techniques of Cognitive Behavioral Therapy* (pp. 640-647). Hoboken, NJ: John Wiley and Sons Inc.

Koegel, Robert L, Openden, Daniel, and Koegel, Lynn Kern 2004. A systematic desensitization paradigm to treat hypersensitivity to auditory stimuli in children with autism in family contexts. *Research and Practice for Persons with Severe Disabilities, 29*(2), 122-124. doi: https://doi.org/10.2511/rpsd.29.2.122.

Lucker, Jay R 2013. Auditory hypersensitivity in children with autism spectrum disorder. *Focus on Autism and Other Developmental Disabilities, 28*(3), 184-191. doi: https://doi.org/10.1177/1088357 613475810.

Lucker, Jay R. 2014a. Auditory Processing Disorders in Children with Autism Spectrum Disorders. *Autism Notebook, April 2014 issue*.

Lucker, Jay R. 2014b. *What Are Auditory Processing Disorders Really All About.* Electronic publication available online at www.special-ism.org.

Lucker, Jay R. 2014c. *Evaluating the Different Types of Auditory Processing Deficits.* Electronic publication available on line at www.special-ism.org.

Lucker, Jay R. 2014d. *Treatments for Different Types of Auditory Processing Deficits.* Electronic publication available online at www.special-ism.org.

Lucker, Jay R. 2018a. Auditory processing: How Does it Really Work? Part 2: A Multisystem Approach. *Hearing Health Matters e-journal,* on-line publication available at: http://hearinghealthmatters.org/theaudiology condition/2018/auditory-processing-how-does-it-really-work-part-2/.

Lucker Jay R. 2018b. Auditory processing: How Does It Really Work? Part 1. *Hearing Health Matters e-journal,* on-line publication available at: http://hearinghealthmatters.org/theaudiologycondition/2018/ auditory-processing-how-does-it-really-work/.

Lucker Jay R and Doman Alex 2012. Auditory hypersensitivity and autism spectrum disorder: An emotional response. *Autism Science Digest: The Journal of Autismone, 4*, 103-108.

Lucker Jay R. and Doman, Alex. 2015. Neural mechanisms involved in hypersensitive hearing: Helping children with ASD who are overly sensitive to sounds. *Autism Research and Treatment, 215*, 1-8. doi: http://dx.doi.org/10.1155/2015/369035.

Lucker Jay R and Doman, Alex. 2019. Use of acoustically modified music to reduce auditory hypersensitivities in children. *Sound and Listening in Health Care Therapy. Music and Medicine, 11* (1), 48-54.

Moller, Aage R, and Rollins, Pamela Rosenthal (2002). The non-classical auditory pathways are involved in hearing in children but not adults.

*Neuroscience Letters, 19* (1), 41-44. doi: 10.1016/s0304-3940(01) 02516-2.

Moller, Aage R, Kern, Janet K, and Grannemann, Bruce 2005. Are the non-classical auditory pathways involved in autism and PDD? *Neurological Research, 27*(6), 625-629. doi: 10.1179/016164105X25117.

Occupational Safety and Health Administration n.d. *How Loud is Too Loud?* Accessed November 30, 2019. https://www.osha.gov/SLTC/noisehearingconservation/loud.html.

Porges, Stephen W 2011. The polyvagal theory: New insights into adaptive reactions of the autonomic nervous system. *Cleveland Clinical Journal of Medicine, 76* (2), S86-S90. doi: 10.3949/ccjm.76.s2.17.

Reeves, Christa and Lucker Jay R. 2017. Analysis of changes in auditory processing after therapy. *Topics in Central Auditory Processing, 2* (3), 6-9.

Stiegler, Lillian N and Davis, Rebecca 2010. Understanding sound sensitivity in individuals with autism spectrum disorder. *Focus on Autism and Other Developmental Disabilities, 25*(2), 67-75. doi: https//doi.org/10.1177/1088357610364530.

Vargas, Sadako and Lucker, Jay R. (2016). A Quantitative Summary of The Listening Program (TLP) Efficacy Studies: What Areas were found to improve by TLP intervention? *Occupational Therapy International*. [Available in print in journal an "early view" online at: http://onlinelibrary.wiley.com/doi/10.1002/oti.1425/full.

## BIOGRAPHICAL SKETCH

### *Jay R. Lucker*

**Affiliation:** Department of Communication Sciences and Disorders, Howard University, Washington, DC - also – Certified/Licensed Audiologist and Speech-Language Pathologist specializing in Auditory and Language Processing Disorders with Part-Time Private Practice in the Greater Washington DC area.

**Education:** EdD in Audiology and Auditory Neuroscience from Columbia University in New York City; Master's Degree (MA) in Audiology from Hunter College of the City University of New York and in Speech-Language Pathology from Lehman College of the City University of New York; Bachelor's Degree (BA) in Speech-Language Pathology and Audiology from Hunter College in the Bronx of the City University of New York

**Research and Professional Experience:** Multiple presentations, mostly invited presentations, internationally in the area of auditory processing both concepts about auditory processing, how to evaluate auditory processing, interpretation of auditory processing test results, evidence-based treatments for auditory processing disorders and language processing problems in children and adolescents. I am a research specialist in the areas of auditory processing and language processing primarily in children and adolescents.

**Professional Appointments:** Professor at Howard University; Adjunct Professor at Rocky Mountain University of Health Professions in Provo, UT (I teach on-line/distance learning course in Practice Management for Speech-Language Pathology)

**Honors:** American Academy of Audiology – Honors of the association; Honors from the New York City Speech-Language-Hearing Association for professional contributions to the area.

**Publications from the Last 3 Years:**

*Articles*

1) Lucker, J (2019). Can children with auditory processing disorders receive services in schools. *Topics in Central Auditory Processing*, 3(6), 2-5.

2) Lucker J, Doman A (2019). Use of acoustically modified music to reduce auditory hypersensitivities in children. *Sound and Listening in Health Care Therapy. Music and Medicine, 11* (1).
3) Lucker, JR, Chang J, Finley N, Mims A, Silva A. (2018). What Do Non-Verbal Measures of Auditory Processing Tell Us? *Topics in Central Auditory Processing, 3* (4), 7-11.
4) Lucker JR, Molloy AT (2018). What Parents of Children with Chromosome Variations Feel About Special Education Teacher's Understanding of Their Children's Educational Problems. *Special Education Research, Policy, & Practice, 2* (1), 45-53.
5) Lucker, JR, Lindsay K, Toogood S, Hawkins J, Edwards-Gaither L, Khabo B, Harris DJ (2018). At What Age Should We Test for Auditory Processing Disorders? Results of Professional and Parent Surveys. *Topics in Central Auditory Processing, 3* (3), 6-10.
6) Lucker JR (2018). Auditory processing: How Does it Really Work? Part 2: A Multisystem Approach. *Hearing Health Matters e-journal,* on-line publication available at: http://hearinghealthmatters.org/theaudiologycondition/2018/auditory-processing-how-does-it-really-work-part-2/.
7) Lucker JR (2018). Auditory processing: How Does It Really Work? Part 1. *Hearing Health Matters e-journal,* on-line publication available at: http://hearinghealthmatters.org/theaudiology condition/2018/auditory-processing-how-does-it-really-work/.
8) Lucker JR (2018). Evidence supports testing children younger than age 7 for auditory processing disorders. *The Hearing Review, 25*(4), 42.
9) Chakraborty S, Kaf W, Lucker JR (2018). Interactive Metronome: Research review related to treating auditory processing disorders in children. *Journal of the Academy of Rehabilitative Audiology, XLX,* 1-9.
10) Hawkins J, Lucker JR (2018). Auditory processing disorders: A unifying definition and professional implications. *Topics in Central Auditory Processing, 3*(1), 5-9.

11) Kaul K, Lucker JR (2017). Analyzing SIR for integration weakness. *Topics in Central Auditory Processing, 2* (4), 2-6.
12) Lucker J (2017). School policies regarding children with auditory processing disorders. *Special Education Research, Policy and Practice, 1* (1), 138-145.
13) Lucker J (2017). Auditory processing testing: In the booth versus outside the booth. *Journal of the American Academy of Audiology (JAAA), 28* (1), 1-6.
14) Reeves C, Lucker JR (2017). Analysis of changes in auditory processing after therapy. *Topics in Central Auditory Processing, 2* (3), 6-9.
15) Safi M, Wright-Harp W, Lucker JR, Payne JC (2017). Effect of neuromuscular electrical stimulation on labial and lingual muscles in healthy volunteers. *International Journal of Rehabilitation Research, 40* (2), 119-126.
16) Safi M, Wright-Harp W, Lucker, JR, Payne JC (2017). Effect of neuromuscular electrical stimulation on labial and lingual weakness: A single-case prexperimental study. *Topics in Geriatric Rehabilitation.*
17) Lucker, J.R. (2017, July). Auditory processing disorder is a legitimate clinical entity. *The ASHA Leader, 22*(4). Available on line: http://leader.pubs.asha.org/article.aspx?articleid=2643064.
18) Lucker, J.R. (2017, February). Testing young children for APD. *The ASHA Leader, 22*(1). Available on line: http://leader.pubs.asha.org/article.aspx?articleid=2600873&resultClick=3.

*Book Chapters*

1) Lucker JR (2018). How Auditory Processing Deficits Can Interfere with a College Student's Success in School and Work. (Chapter 35). In M Valente & ML Valente (editors). *Adult Audiology Casebook,* Second Edition. NY: Thieme Publishers. Also available on-line at: https://medone-comsic.thieme.com/cockpits/claudiology/0/coCPeComCa0335/0.

2) Lucker JR (2018). Hearing versus Auditory Processing Disorders: Are Hearing Aids Enough? (Chapter 36). In M Valente & ML Valente (editors). *Adult Audiology Casebook*, Second Edition. NY: Thieme Publishers. Also available on-line at: https://medone-comsic.thieme.com/cockpits/claudiology/0/coCPeComCa0336/0.
3) Lucker JR (2018). Auditory Processing Disorders. In D. Geffner & D. Ross-Swain (Editors), *Auditory Processing Disorders in Children: Assessment, Management, and Treatment*, Third Edition. San Diego, CA: Plural Publishing.

*Invited Professional Presentations (last three years)*

1) Lucker JR, Kaul K (2019, September). Integrating auditory-speech-language systems and other processes. *Invited presentation made for continuing education credit at the 2019 Annual Conference of the International Guild of Auditory Processing Specialists*, Kansas City, MO.
2) Lucker JR (2019, May). Auditory Processing Testing in Children: Providing Meaningful Interpretation and Recommendations. *Invited presentation made for continue education credit at the 2019 Spring Conference of the California Audiology Association*, San Jose, CA.
3) Lucker JR (2019, April). Assessing Auditory Processing Disorders in Children: Appropriate Evaluations and Interpretation. *Invited presentation made for continuing education credit at the 2019 Annual Convention of the Missouri Speech-Language-Hearing Association*, Ozark Lake, Missouri.
4) Lucker JR (2019, April). Appropriate evidence-Based treatments for auditory processing disorders same as above. *Invited presentation made for continuing education credit at the 2019 Annual Convention of the Missouri Speech-Language-Hearing Association*, Ozark Lake, Missouri.
5) Lucker, JR (2019, April). Evidence Based Evaluation and Treatment for Children with Auditory Processing Disorders. *Invited presentation for continuing education credit made at the 2019*

*Annual Convention of the National Black Association for Speech, Language, and Hearing*, Charlotte, NC.

6) Lucker, JR (2019, April). Speech Science for the Praxis. *Invited presentation for the Praxis Review Course presented at the 2019 Annual Convention of the National Black Association for Speech, Language, and Hearing, Charlotte, NC.*
7) Lucker, JR (2019, April). Professional Issues, Ethics and Research for the Praxis. *Invited presentation for the Praxis Review Course presented at the 2019 Annual Convention of the National Black Association for Speech, Language, and Hearing, Charlotte, NC.*
8) Lucker JR (2019, April). Understanding Auditory Processing Disorders: What Psychologists Need to Know. *Invited presentation made at the Chicago School for Professional Psychology*, Washington, DC.
9) Lucker JR (2019, March). *Evaluating and interpreting APD test results in an educationally appropriate manner 2019 Annual convention of SHAV March 2019 Richmond VA.*
10) Lucker JR (2019, March). Effective Treatments for Children with Auditory Processing Disorders – Part 1. *Invited presentation for continuing education credit made at the 2019 Annual convention of SHAV March 2019 Richmond VA*.
11) Lucker JR (2019, March). Effective Treatments for Children with Auditory Processing Disorders – Part 2. *Invited presentation for continuing education credit made at the 2019 Annual convention of SHAV March 2019 Richmond VA.*
12) Lucker JR (2019, January). Therapies for Children with Auditory Processing Disorders. *Invited presentation for continuing education credit presented at the Winter 2019 Convention of the Maryland Speech-Language-Hearing Association, Rockville, MD.*
13) Lucker JR (2019, January). Mythbusting Auditory Processing Disorders. *Invited presentation for continuing education credit presented at the Winter 2019 Convention of the Maryland Speech-Language-Hearing Association, Rockville, MD.*

14) Lucker JR (2018, December). Problems Faced by Seniors Hearing What People Say. *Invited Presentation made to the Seniors and Professionals at Good Shepherd Lutheran Church, Gaithersburg,* MD.
*15)* Lucker, JR (2018, September). What are Auditory Processing Disorders Really All About? *Invited presentation presented for continuing education credit from the American Speech-Language-Hearing Association (ASHA) for the Baltimore City Speech-Language Pathology Association*
16) Lucker JR (2018, April). Significance of Qualitative Errors on Auditory Processing Evaluations. *Invited presentation made at the 2018 Semi-Annual Convention of the International Guild of Auditory Processing Specialists (IGAPS). Kansas City, MO.*
17) Kaul K, Lucker JR (2018, April). Effective Therapies for Children with Auditory Processing Disorders. *Invited presentation made at the 2018 Semi-Annual Convention of the International Guild of Auditory Processing Specialists (IGAPS), Kansas City, MO.*
18) Lucker JR (2018, April). Professional Practice and Ethics. *Invited course presented for the PRAXIS REVIEW at the 2018 Annual Convention of the National Black Association for Speech, Language, and Hearing (NBASLH), Crystal City, VA.*
*19)* Lucker, JR (2018, April). Speech Science. *Invited course presented for the PRAXIS REVIEW at the 2018 Annual Convention of the National Black Association for Speech, Language, and Hearing (NBASLH), Crystal City, VA.*
20) Lucker JR (2018, April). Appropriate Therapies for Children with Different Types of Auditory Processing Disorders. *Invited presentation at the 2018 Annual Convention of the Maryland Speech-Language-Hearing Association, Annapolis, MD.*
21) Lucker JR (2017, April). Stats 101 – Analyzing Your Data. *Invited presentation made at the 2017 Annual Convention of the International Guild of Auditory Processing Specialists (IGAPS).* Kansas City, MO.

*22)* Lucker, J.R. (2017, April). Speech Science Praxis Review Course. *Invited course presentation made at the 2017 Annual Convention of the National Black Association for Speech, Language, and Hearing (NBASLH), Nashville, TN.*

23) Lucker, J.R. (2017, April). Ethics and Professional Practice Praxis Review Course. *Invited course presentation made at the 2017 Annual Convention of the National Black Association for Speech, Language, and Hearing (NBASLH), Nashville, TN.*

24) Lucker, JR (2017, March). Understanding Auditory Processing Disorders in Children, *Invited short course (one full day) made at the 2017 Annual Convention of the North Carolina Speech-Language-Hearing Association.*

In: Understanding Children with Autism … ISBN: 978-1-53617-647-6
Editor: Anne Bourque 

*Chapter 2*

# UNDERSTANDING HEARING LOSS IN CHILDREN WITH AUTISM SPECTRUM DISORDER

***Annette E. Hurley*** * ***and Sloane C. Henry***
Department of Communication Disorders,
Louisiana State University Health Sciences Center,
New Orleans, Louisiana

## ABSTRACT

Hearing loss is the most common developmental abnormality present at birth in approximately two to four per 1000 newborns (Fitzpatrick, Lambert, Whittingham & Leblanc, 2014; Prieve & Stevens, 2000). The negative effects of undiagnosed hearing loss include delayed language, learning, and speech development. Approximately 40% of children with hearing loss will have an accompanying disorder according to a recent epidemiological report by Gallaudet Research Institute in 2009 (Meinzen-Derr, Wiley, Bishop, Manning-Courtney, Choo & Murray, 2013). Autism Spectrum Disorder (ASD) is a common neurodevelopmental disorder, which also negatively affects

* Corresponding Author's E-mail: ahurle@lsuhsc.edu.

communication and social interaction. Interestingly, the prevalence of ASD in the general population is 1 in 68 but rises to 1 in 59 in children with hearing loss (Szymanski, Brice, Lam, & Hotto, 2012). The chapter will highlight the relationship between ASD and hearing loss and the challenges associated with making a dual diagnosis. It will discuss specific anatomical differences in the central auditory pathway and brain, the auditory processing of acoustic stimuli in children with ASD, and the audiological management of children with ASD, including hypersensitivity.

**Keywords:** hearing loss, auditory processing, autism spectrum disorder

## INTRODUCTION

Hearing loss affects two to four newborns per 1000 births (Fitzpatrick, Lambert, Whittingham & Leblanc, 2014; Prieve & Stevens, 2000) and of those identified, an estimated 40% will most likely have an accompanying developmental disability (Meinzen-Derr, Wiley, Bishop, Manning-Courtney, Choo & Murray, 2013; Fitzpatrick et al., 2014). It is important for audiologists to recognize possible red flags for other accompanying disabilities so that a proper referral to other disciplines or a multi-disciplinary team can be made in order for appropriate intervention to begin as soon as possible.

Autism Spectrum Disorder (ASD) is a range of neurodevelopmental disorders that affect people on an individual basis, with great variability (American Psychiatric Association, 2013). ASD is multifactorial in etiology and can vary in severity and functionality per the individual. Diagnosis criteria set forth by the Diagnostic and Statistical Manual of Mental Disorders V (DSM-V) includes two major defining characteristics integrated with all sub-diagnoses: social communication/interaction and restricted, repetitive behaviors (Hyman, 2013). The chapter will further highlight the relationship between ASD and hearing loss and the challenges associated with making a dual diagnosis. It will discuss specific anatomical differences in the central auditory pathway, the processing ability of incoming stimuli in children with ASD, and the audiological management of children with ASD, including hypersensitivity.

## HEARING LOSS AND AUTISM SPECTRUM DISORDER: A DUAL DIAGNOSIS

Autism Spectrum Disorder (ASD) negatively affects children in the areas of communication and social interactions, with additional characterizations of repetitive and restrictive behavioral patterns. Similarly, permanent hearing loss negatively affects children in areas of communication, speech and language development, and in some cases social abilities. The prevalence of ASD in the general population is 1 in 68 but rises to 1 in 59 in children with hearing loss (Szymanski, Brice, Lam, & Hotto, 2012). ASD and hearing loss, when identified individually, constitute a large proportion of children in the general population. Delays in communication, which are often associated with ASD, may be attributed to the hearing loss itself. Although ASD and hearing loss share similar behavioral charteristics, they are distinct conditions.

Characterizing a comorbid diagnosis is challenging, since delays in language and communication are symptoms of both hearing loss and ASD. Although a challenge, the importance of identification of these two separate, comorbid diagnoses is critical in initiating the proper intervention services in order to promote language and communication skills. ASD is increasing in prevalence due to awareness and access to services and is now one of the most diagnosed developmental disorders in children. It is important for children diagnosed with ASD to have an audiological assessment to rule out any degree of hearing loss.

There are two main types of hearing loss. One type, conductive hearing loss, results from abnormalities in the external or middle ear. Previous investigations have reported an increased number of occurrences of conductive losses due to otitis media (ear infections) in the ASD population compared to typically normal peers (Konstantareas, Homatidis, 1987; Rosenhall, Nordin, Sandstrom, Ahlsen & Gillberg, 1999; Smith, Miller, Stewart, Walter & McConnell, 1988). Smith et al. (1988) observed more instances of abnormal negative middle ear pressure occurring in children with ASD compared to a control group, during a a 10-week study.

The second type of hearing loss is sensorineural hearing loss. This type of hearing loss occurs from damage in the inner ear, cochlea or auditory nerve. A recent epidemiological report from Gallaudet Research Institute (2006) reported 1 in 59 children with hearing loss would also be diagnosed with ASD; an incidence rate higher than the general population (Szymanski et al., 2012). In instances of dual diagnoses of hearing loss and ASD, the identification of a hearing loss is usually obtained first (Fitzpatrick et al., 2014, Roper, Arnold & Monteiro 2003; Szymanski et al., 2012; Worley et al., 2011). Meinzen-Derr et al. (2014) report the average age of diagnosis of hearing loss was 14 months, while the average age for a diagnosos of ASD was significantly delayed to 66.5 months. The degree of hearing loss can range from a mild to a profound degree and there are a variety of audiometric configurations. Additionally, investigations have reported that the diagnosis of ASD in children with severe to profound hearing loss is more difficult to make because of the communication delays that are attributed to the significant degree of hearing loss.

However, Meinzen-Derr et al. (2014) report that children with a severe to profound hearing loss who underwent cochlear implantation received a diagnosis of ASD earlier than children with a moderate or mild degree of hearing loss. The authors attributed this to the fact that these children were engaged in follow up evaluations for cochlear implantation. Clinicians may have been alerted to red flags or other delays that exceeded those of a typical hearing impaired child's performance post implantation, and therefore made the proper referral for diagnosis (Meinzen-Derr et al., 2014).

It is important to note that an inaccuracy of diagnoses can occur. Kozlowski, Matson & Horovitz (2011) report children misdiagnosed with ASD, rather than an organic hearing loss, and children with ASD incorrectly diagnosed with hearing loss. Therefore, it is extremely important to differentiate these disorders. Currently, the diagnosis of ASD is based upon a child's developmental progress including social and communication development, which again could be affected with any degree of hearing loss.

The earlier a diagnosis is made, the earlier that intervention can begin. However, it is likely a hearing loss will be diagnosed first. This is in part due to the initiatives set forth in the Early Hearing Detection and Intervention

(EDHI) programs (Joint Commision on Infant Hearing, 2019). In summary, all newborns will have a diagnosis of hearing loss by 3 months of age with intervention beginning by 6 moths of age. It is important to note that a newborn hearing screening does not detect mild hearing loss, or hearing loss that is acquired after birth due to infections, or a progressive hearing loss.

## Importance of Differential Diagnosis

As noted, early diagnosis and intervention is crucial in the acquisition and development of language and communication abilities in children. Thus, the identification of any disorder that could potentially delay or halt such development is of critical importance. Since many characteristic symptoms of ASD can mimic the symptoms present in children with a hearing loss, and vice versa, Worley, Matson, & Kozlowski (2011) sought to highlight the importance in distinguishing hearing loss from ASD in children. These investigators identified communication and socialization impairments as the two main overlapping symptoms common to both children with ASD and children with hearing loss. Worleyet al. (2011) compared the symptomology of 74 children with hearing loss or ASD. The authors caution using communication deficits as a diagnostic criteria for either ASD or hearing loss, as deficits in communication and language are present in both conditions. Clinicians should not let a communication deficit define or take precedence over impairments in areas of socialization and/or repetitive behaviors characteristics, when evaluating for ASD or hearing loss in children. Burns, Matson, Vervantes, Jiang, & Estabillo (2016) note the resulting communication deficits from ASD and hearing loss, although present similarly, stem from two different places of origin. In individuals with hearing loss, communication impairments tend to result from a delayed language development model. While in individuals with ASD, impairments are attributed to an atypical language development model. In support, communication impairments should not be the sole deficit that differentially diagnoses hearing loss from ASD. Some differences noted in communication characteristics of typical children with ASD and children with hearing loss are briefly described in Table 1.

**Table 1. Typical Behaviors for ASD and Hearing Loss**

| | ASD | Hearing Loss |
|---|---|---|
| Social Communication | Atypical eye contact<br>Limited social interaction | Appropriate social smile<br>Appropriate eye contact<br>Appropriate reciprocal behavior<br>Engages in their environment |
| Interactive Communication | Abnormalities in body language<br>Limited facial expressions and gestures<br>Difficulties in non-verbal language | Appropriate eye contact<br>Wide range of gestures<br>Language learning will follow sequence as typical peers<br>May have some difficulty with vocabulary, grammar, or other idiomatic expressions |
| Repetitive Speech | Repetitive speech (i.e., echolalia or idiosyncratic language) | Typically follows normal language development<br>Echolalia occurs only as a developmental stage, does not continue. |

## Assessment and Management of Children with ASD and Hearing Loss

With the implementation of universal newborn hearing screening, mandated by EHDI programs, often a moderate or greater degree degree of hearing loss is identified shortly after birth and early intervention can begin. According to JCIH Position Statement (2019), a child should have an audiological assessment any time there is parent or caregiver concern regarding the child's hearing, speech or language delay or language regression. In addition, an audiological diagnostic assessment is recommended before the child is 3 months of age if the child has passed a newborn hearing screening, but has any of the following risk factors:

- In utero infection with cytomegalovirus (CMV)
- Any event associated with hearing loss such as head trauma or chemotherapy
- Prolonged mechanical ventilation
- Bacterial or viral meningitis or encephalitis.

An audiological follow-up before 9 months of age is recommended for children with the following risk factors:

- Family history of congenital or delayed-onset childhood sensorineural impairment
- Neonatal intensive care for more than 5 days
- Hyperbilirubinemia requiring exchange transfusion
- Ototoxic medications used for more than 5 days
- Severe asphyxia
- Craniofacial anomalies.

Pediatric audiologists are skilled to assess uncooperative children and face many challenges in obtaining frequency specific auditory information. It is imperative that they effectively test and adapt to the challenges that are often faced during testing. There are many reasons it is difficult to test a child with ASD. This could be due to cognitive dysfunction, inattentiveness, increased anxiety, intolerance to earphones, difficulty with following instructions, or difficulty in adapting to new situations (Rosenhall et al., 1999).

Pediatric audiologists are skilled to evaluate hearing on difficult-to-test populations. Often testing a child with ASD may be similar to testing a developmentally delayed individual. Tests or protocols may require modifications and/or special accommodations. It is still necessary to obtain accurate information so that intervention can begin as soon as possible. As previously mentioned, children with hearing loss present with similar symptoms as those who may have ASD, and hearing loss is usually diagnosed first. With this said, audiologists may be the first clinicians to see children in this specific population and need to be aware of other red flags.

Poor eye contact, reduced language comprehension, limited use of gestures, delayed speech with no babbling, and unusual verbalizations are a few behaviors that are commonly seen or reported by the caregivers at the initial appointment (Szarkowski & Johnston, 2018). These behaviors make differentially diagnosing hearing loss from ASD challenging. According to Szarkowski & Johnston (2018) poor eye contact and reduced comprehension are related to ASD and hearing loss in two different ways. Poor eye contact in children with ASD stems from social cognition deficits, while in children with hearing loss, poor eye contact results when children struggle to comprehend spoken language and they no longer attend to the speaker's face. Reduced language comprehension, in children with hearing loss may be the result of insufficient or limited access to incoming auditory stimuli, whereas in children with ASD it is most likely due to cognitive deficits.

With the overlap in symptomology, most caregivers are quick to ask if these developmental deficits are caused by hearing loss and are seen by an audiologist prior to seeking any additional diagnoses (Madell, 2014). If this is the case, and no pre-existing disorder, such as ASD has been diagnosed, it is up to the audiologist to make the proper referrals. Though, it is not up to the audiologist to diagnose ASD, it is still within their scope of practice and is their responsibility to have an understanding of the disorder and be able to recognize the signs and symptoms, along with any effect on hearing, in order to refer and manage accordingly (Madell, 2014). If the opposite is the case, and a child already has a previous diagnosis of ASD, it is also the responsibility of the audiologist to properly and effectively evaluate the child, diagnose and manage any hearing loss, and be an additional member of the child's multidisciplinary team (Madell, 2014).

## Audiological Assessment

The goal of audiological assessment is to obtain threshold information, the lowest intensity level heard by an individual at frequencies important for communication for the right and left ears. These responses are subject to participant cooperation, task comprehension, and behavioral response in order to provide a valid estimate of hearing function. Pediatric audiologists will usually employ both objective and subjective tests in order to obtain information.

The case history is one of the most invaluable pieces of the evaluation process for the audiologist. It allows the clinician to gain insight into the child's history from birth to present day and any other present diagnoses that may halt or warrant modifications of the testing protocol. It prefaces the evaluation and allows the clinician to be on the lookout for any non-typical characteristics or note the presence of one in the absence of any parental concern. Specific questions about speech and language development are included and offer important information to the clinician. When assessing a child with ASD for hearing loss it is important to identify their cognitive age in order to most efficiently obtain audiometric results (Madell, 2014). This information allows clinicians to perform the evaluation using protocols most suitable to the child's needs and abilities.

A comprehensive audiological assessment will include several different tests to assess different anatomical parts of the ear and auditory pathway. The order of the tests may change due to the cooperation and tolerance of a child. Normally, the audiologist would likely use an otoscope to ensure a clear ear canal. The use of insert earphones, headphones or other ear canal probe tips used in audiometric assessment may be uncomforatble for a child who is sensitive to having someone touch his or her ears. Table 2 lists the audiological tests commonly used during an audiological assessment.

Clinicians and parents can do several things to prepare the child for the appointment. Parents or caregivers are an essential part of the assessment. Prior to the appointment, the clinician may inquire about the child's likes and dislikes and have toys that are of his/her favorite interest available. The clinical sight could be send informational pictures, brochures, or stories of what will happen during the testing session. Parents may begin playing "hearing games" at home and have the child wear headphones to begin to tolerate headphones. It may be necessary to have the child visit the booth, or conduct a case history in the testing booth. This will allow the child to acclimate to the testing environment before conducting otoscopy, tympanometry or otoacoustic emissions, (all tests that require having their ears touched). It is necessary and extremely important for clinicians to take extra time to establish a positive rapport when assessing a child with ASD.

**Table 2. Audiological Test Battery**

| Test | Description |
|---|---|
| Otoscopy | Visualization to ensure clear auditory canals and normal appearing tympanic membrane |
| Tympanometry | Middle Ear assessment (Tympanic membrane movement) |
| Pure Tone Audiometry | Auditory threshold information in the frequency range from 250 -8000 Hz, the frequency range important for speech |
| Visual Reinforcement Audiometry | A conditioning method used for young children, requires a child to localize to a sound source. The child is rewarded by animation/lights. |
| Conditioned Play Audiometry | Auditory thresholds are obtained by ‘playing a game’; a child responds by putting a toy in a box, or other “fun” task after he hears a sound. |
| Otoacoustic Emission Test | A relatively quick objective measure of hearing. A small probe, which contains a microphone, is placed in the child’s ear. Sounds are presented through the probe and a response from the cochlea travels back through the middle ear and is picked up by the microphone. This test is often used for hearing screening. |
| Auditory Brainstem Response (ABR) | This is an objective measure of the auditory pathway’s response to sound. Electrodes are placed on the child’s head. A variety of frequency-specific sounds are presented, and a response is obtained. The child should be very quiet during this test. Sedation may be suggested in order to get definitive results. |

The audiologist will obtain frequency specific information about the child’s hearing for each ear. This may be completed by a screening process or adaptable procedures such as visual reinforcement audiometry or conditioned play audiometry. The audiologist may begin to test one low (500 Hz) and mid-frequency (2000Hz) pure tone. Children with ASD may not respond well to speech stimuli. If a hearing loss is suspected and results cannot be obtained by behavioral measures, the child may be referred for an auditory brainstem response test (ABR). The ABR is a neural synchronous response from the auditory nerve and lower brainstem. The ABR should be obtained when the child is quiet; therefore, this may require sedation.

Additional tests will often be administered, if possible, during the initial appointment. Tympanometry is an objective test of the middle ear function.

This test will show how the tympanic membrane moves and will provide information on how well the Eustachian tube is working to ventilate the middle ear space. The audiologist may also obtain information from the outer hair cells of the cochlea by recording otoacoustic emissions (OAEs). OAEs provide frequency specific information and may be used as a hearing screener. However, it is important to note that both tympanometry and OAE testing requires a small probe to be inserted into the ear canal. Often, children with ASD may be very sensitive to having anything in their ears and these tests may be completed after pure-tone behavioral testing has been completed.

## Management

If a hearing loss is present, the child will be fit with amplification. The hearing aids should be appropriately programmed to provide the necessary amount of gain for each frequency. It is also important for the child to have consistent use of hearing technology. Wearing the hearing aids daily will provide the best access to audibility. Providing amplification to a child with ASD will also promote language acquisition and development. However, the potential outcomes for auditory development will be variable. Spoken language may not always be the outcome, even if a child has a cochlear implant or well-aided hearing. It is important for the clinician to discuss realistic expectations from amplification. Further, an augmentative and alternative communication device assessment by a speech-language pathologist may be warranted.

When evaluating and managing a child for hearing loss, it is common for those with ASD (pre or post diagnosis) to experience a fear of noise. Hypersensitivity or hyperacusis is a heightened or abnormal sensitivity to sound. This may due to the abnormal brain differences that will be described in a later section. Gravel, Dunn, Lee & Ellis (2006) and Tharpe et al. (2006) report that children with ASD do not have more sensitive hearing than their typical peers. However, parents of children with ASD report increased anxiety or distress when exposed to certain sound, avoidance and other negative reactions or uncomfortable sensations related to some sounds (Koegel & Koegel, 2006). Some of these behaviors include but are not limited to, crying, hitting, or "shutting down", when there is too much auditory stimulation (Madell, 2014). In these cases, it is important to have careful control over the loud stimuli presented during testing and introduce it only when the child's attention has decreased to re-alert and re- focus their attention, without alarming them (Madell, 2014). It is also important that concise descriptions of the sounds that are most bothersome to the child are reported during the audiologcial case history.

In addition to hearing aids, assistive listening devices (ALDs) can be utilized to enhance the child's listening ability. Specifically, the use of frequency modulated (FM) or remote microphone (RM) systems have proven to significantly improve the speech scores as well as increase attention and on-task behaviors in the classroom for children with ASD and hearing loss (Schafer et al., 2012). The FM or RM system will improve the signal to noise ratio for the listener. Specifically, Schafer et al. (2012) report a significant reduction in two specific behaviors when children with a dual diagnosis utilized an FM system: a reduction in the children's inability to follow teacher direction and their inability to sit quietly when asked of them. There was also a reduction in the amount of distractible classroom behaviors that the children engaged in (i.e., out of seat, blurts out answers without raising hands, playing with anything in hands or with hands, shaking head back and forth) (Schafer et al., 2012).

## Anatomical Brain Differences and Auditory Processing

There is ample evidence from the scientific literature reporting brain differences in those with ASD compared to typical brains. Structural differences occur in many different parts of the brain, including the auditory and auditory processing centers of the brain. Several structural and functional neurobiological abnormalities may contribute to the sensory processing impairments exhibited by children with ASD. Several regions of the brain of children with ASD show abnormalities including differences in head circumference, frontal lobe hyperplasia (an excess of cells or tissue), abnormal cortical organization, abnormal minicolumn structure in frontal and temporal areas, and variations in white and gray matter and sensory deficits (Gerrard & Rugg, 2009). There are also reports of abnormalities in the gray matter brainstem (Jou et al., 2009) and abnormalities in the cerebellum (Iarocci & McDonald, 2005). There are also differences in regard to neural transmission including synaptogenesis (the formation of synapses, especially important during key periods of brain development), neural pruning (a neurological regulatory process that produces a more efficient synaptic configuration by reducing the number of neurons) and myelination (the wrapping of neurons in myelin, which allows rapid transmission of neuronal signals) (Gerrard & Rugg, 2009). There are also differences reported in the superior olivary complex. The superior olivary complex is very important in auditory processing, as this is the place where binaural information occurs. This structure is also important in localization and hearing in background noise. Researchers have found the superior olivary complex to be smaller in individuals with ASD (Kulesza, Lukose & Stevens 2011).

Another brain structure important in auditory processing is the corpus callosum (CC). The CC is a body of neural fibers that connects the right and left hemisphere and allows for integration of information between the two hemispheres. Previous investigations have shown deficits in the size of the corpus callosum in children with autism (Chung et al., 2004; Egaas, Courchesne, Saitoh, 1995; Haas et al., 1996; Manes et al., 1999; Waiter et al., 2005). Different regions of the CC have specialized sensory functions. The posterior portion or the isthumus is specialized for auditory information. Thus, abnormalities of cortical connectivity lead to a disruption of integrative processing.

The ABR reflects synchronous firing of the auditory nerve and lower brainstem. This test may be used to obtain frequency specific information for patients who do not respond behaviorally. Miron, Beam, and Kohane (2018) completed a meta-analysis of the ABR response in children with

ASD. They report a longer response in those with ASD than typical brains. Reasons for this delay could be due to brain overgrowth in children with ASD (Courchesne et al., 20011) or an increase in head circumference size (Mitchell, Phillips & Trune, 1989). Additionally, differences in myelination may result in slower neural conduction, thus affecting wave latencies. Russo, Nicol, Trommel, Zecker & Kraus (2008) reported prolonged latencies and reduced amplitudes in the speech ABR recorded in quiet and in noise in a group of children with ASD compared to typical children. These authors conclude that abnormalities in the brainstem that encode the speech signal are responsible in part for language impairments in the ASD population.

The P300 is a cortical response and reflects activity from the auditory cortex. It is is an endogenous response, indicating the listener responds to changes in the auditory the stimulus. Cui, Wang, Liu, Zhang (2017) published a meta-analysis of the P300 response in individuals with ASD and report prolonged latencies and reduced amplitudes of the P300 response for individuals with ASD. The authors attribute these differences in the P300 response may reflect attention, working memory, or other informational processing ability.

Otoacousic emissions are responses generated by the outer hair cells of the cochlea. Khalfa et al. (2001) reported a decrease in transient evoked otoacoustic emission (TEOAE) amplitudes for children with ASD but not for typically developing peers, possibly suggesting a premature deterioration of outer hair cell function.

Abnormalities have also been reported for the efferent auditory system in individuals with ASD. In humans, the medial olivochohlear (MOC) reflex has been investigated using recordings of OAEs during the simultaneous presentation of contralateral broadband noise TEOAE recordings (Berlin, Hood, Hurley, & Wen, 1994). Several investigations have reported redueced suppression in individuals with ASD (Bennetto, Keith, Allen, & Luebka, 2018; Khalfa et al., 2001). These differences may contribute to some of the auditory processing complaints in individuals with ASD such as hearing in background noise.

Further, Wilson, Sadler, Hancock, Guinan & Lichtenhan (2017) reported a stong correlation between the amount of efferent suppression and hyperacusis. This is the first objective way to possibly identify individuals with hyperacusis.

## Auditory Processing and ASD

A variety of auditory impairments are possible among individuals with ASD. Auditory complaints in children with ASD may be regarded as part of the high-order cognitive disorder and referrals to audiologists, the professionals qualified to treat auditory issues, are not offered or suggested. Children with ASD display atypical auditory processing and demonstrate difficulty tolerating noisy environments, distractibility from listening tasks, distractibility by noise, inability to process lengthy auditory inputs, excessive or abnormal reactions to some loud sounds, and inability to understand or respond to speech. Auditory remediation may be useful and improve communication and increased auditory output in children diagnosed with ASD.

Of interest in the auditory processing disorder assessment is the inclusion of dichotic listening tasks. Dichotic listening tasks are routinely used to assess interhemispheric function (Musiek & Pinheiro, 1985). Dichotic listening refers to the simultaneous presentation of a different auditory signal to each individual ear and reflects interhemispheric function. In normal listening conditions, auditory information is conducted to the auditory cortex by both ipsilateral and contralateral pathways. Most people are left hemisphere language dominant. Thus, the auditory signal from the more numerous, contralateral right auditory pathway is conducted directly to the left hemisphere. The auditory signal directed to the left ear is conducted to the right cortex and must be transferred to the left hemisphere via the corpus callosum. It is not surprising that there is a slight right ear advantage for normal, right-handed listeners when listening to dichotic tasks (Kimura, 1961). Left ear deficits, or unusual right ear deficits are common for children with ASD; however, there can be much improvement after auditory remediation (Denman, Hurley, Banajee, 2015).

There is substantial research that supports the plasticity of the central auditory nervous system and reorganization after auditory training. Because the brain retains a lifelong capacity for plasticity and adaptive reorganization, reorganization may be at least partially reversible through a deficit specific training program. Reorganization is reflected in an increase in the number of synapses, increased neural density, and improvement in electrophysiological recordings and behavioral responses (Elbert antev, Wienbrunch, Rockstroh, & Taub, 1995; Merzenich et al., 1993; Recanzone Schreiner & Merzenich 1993). However, there is a need for investigations to explore auditory processing remediation training in children with ASD.

## Conclusion

Audiologists may be one of the first health care professionals to evaluate a child with ASD due to the communication delays. Hearing loss occurs more often in children with ASD than in the general population. It is important that the audiologist be aware of behaviors that are not consistent with typical pediatric behavioral development and refer when warranted. It is also extremely important for the audiologist to be adaptive in behavioral audiological assessments and recognize the possible need for additional testing sessions in order to obtain accuarate and comprehensive auditory information.

There is a vast number of published studies reporting anatomical brain differences for individuals with ASD when compared to typically developing brains. These structural and functional differences are likely responsible for differences in objective recordings such as the ABR and OAEs and are likely responsible for deficits or differences in auditory processing.

Early identification and enrollment in an intervention program is paramount in a producing a better long-term outcome for children with ASD. Thus, it is crucial that audiologists refer children that they suspect may have ASD based upon parental report and observed behaviors to appropriate professionals. Unfortunately, there is limited research on auditory processing deficits in children with ASD and the success or failure of auditory remedial therapies. We contend that children with ASD may benefit from deficit-specific auditory training consistent with the underlying site of auditory dysfunction.

Although it is beyond the scope of an audiologist to make a diagnosis of ASD, they are often included as part of the multi-disciplinary team, which may do so. Audiologists offer insight into differential diagnosis, helping to determine when there is more than just a hearing loss.

## REFERENCES

Aboitiz, F., Scheibel, A. B., Fisher, R. S. & Zaidel, E. (1992). Fiber composition of human corpus callosum. *Brain Res*, *598*, 143-153.

American Psychiatric Association. (2013). *Diagnostic and statistical manual of mental disorders* (5th ed.) Washington, D.C.

Berlin, C. I., Hood, L. J., Hurley, A. & Wen, H. (1994). Contralateral suppression of otoacoustic emissions: An index of the function of the medial olivocochlear system. *Otolaryngology Head and Neck Surgery. 110*, 3-21.

Burns, C. O., Matson, J. L., Cervantes, P. E., Jiang, X. & Estabillo, J. A. (2016). Hearing impairment, autism spectrum disorder, and developmental functioning in infants and toddlers. *Journal of Developmental & Physical Disabilities*, *284*, 95-507.

Chung, M. K., Robbins, S. M., Dalton, K. M., Davidson, R. J., Alexander, A. L., et al. (2005). Cortical thickness analysis in autism with heat kernel smoothing. *Neuroimage*, *25*, 1256-1265.

Courchesne, E., Mouton, P. R., Calhoun, M. E., Semendeferi, K., Ahrens-Barbeau, C., Hallet, M. J. & Pierce, K. (2011). Neuron number and size in prefrontal cortex of children with autism. *The Journal of the American Medical Association*, *306*, 2001-2010. doi:10.1001/ jama.2011.1638.

Cui, T., Wang, P. P., Liu, S. & Zhang, X. (2017). P300 amplitude and latency in autism spectrum disorder: a meta-analysis *Eur Child Adolesc Psychiatry*, *26*, 177–190DOI 10.1007/s00787-016-0880-z.

Denman, I., Banajee, M. & Hurley, A. (2015). The effect of dichotic listening on children with ASD: A single subject Design. *International Journal of Audiology*, *54*, 991-996.

Elbert, T., Pantev, C., Wienbruch, C., Rockstroh, B. & Taub, E. (1995). Increased use of the left hand in string players associated with increased cortical representation of the fingers. *Science*, *270*, 305–307.

Egaas, B., Courchesne, E. & Saitoh, O. (1995). Reduced size of corpus callosum in autism. *Arch Neurol*, *52*, 794-801.

Fitzpatrick, E. M., Lambert, L., Whittingham, J. & Leblanc, E. (2014). Examination of characteristics and management of children with hearing loss and autism spectrum disorders. *International Journal of Audiology*, *53*, 577-586.

Gallaudet Research Institute. (2006). *Regional and national summary report of data from the 2004 – 2005 Annual Survey of Deaf and Hard of Hearing Children and Youth.* Washington, DC, USA: Gallaudet University.

Gravel, J. S., Dunn, M., Lee, W. W. & Ellis, M. A. (2006). Peripheral audition of children on the autistic spectrum. *Ear Hear*, *27*, 299 – 312.

Haas, R. H., Townsend, J., Courchesne, E., Lincoln, A. J., Schreiban, L. & Yeung-Courchesne, R. (1996). Neurologic abnormalities in infantile autism. *J Child Neurol*, *11*, 84-92.

Hyman, S. L. (2013). New DSM-5 includes changes to autism criteria. *American Academy of Pediatrics.* (doi: 10.1542/ aapnews.20130604-1).

Gallaudet Research Institute. (2009). *Regional and national summary report of data from the 2009-2010 Annual Survey of Deaf and Hard of Hearing Children and Youth.* Washington, DC, USA: Gallaudet University.

Gerrard, S. & Rugg, G. (2009). Sensory impairments and Autism: A Re-Examination of Causal Modeling. *Journal of Autism Dev Discod*, *39*, 1449-1463 doi: 10.1007/s10803-009-0773-9.

Iarocci, G. & McDonald, J. (2006). Sensory Integration and the Perceptual Experiences of Persons with Autism. *Journal of Autism and Developmental Disorders*, *36*, 1, 77-90. Doi:10.1007/s10803-005-0044-3.

Joint Commission on Infant Hearing. (2019). Year 2019 position statement; principles and guidelines for early hearing detection and intervention programs. *The Journal of Early hearing Detection and Intervention*, *4*, 1-44.

Jou, R. J., Minshew, N. J., Melhem, N. M., Keshavan, M. S. & Hardan, A. Y. (2009). Brainstem Volumetric Alterations in Children with autism. *Psychological Medicine*, *39*, 1347-1354. doi: 10.1017/ S0033291 708004376.

Khalfa, S., Bruneau, N., Roge, B., Georgieff, N., Veuillet, E., Adrien, J. & Collet, L. (2001). Peripheral auditory asymmetry in infantile autism. *European Journal of Neuroscience.*, *13*, 628–632.

Kimura, D. (1961). Cerebral dominance and the perception of verbal stimuli. *Canadian Journal of Psychology/Revue canadienne de psychologie*, *15*, 166–171. doi.org/10.1037/h0083219.

Koegel, R. L. & Koegel, L. K. (2006). *Pivotal response treatments for autism: Communication, social, and academic development*. Baltimore, MD: Paul H Brookes Publishing.

Konstantareas, M. & Homatidis, S. (1987). Brief report: ear infections in autistic and normal children. *J Autism Dev Dis*, *17*, 585–593.

Kozlowski, A. M., Matson, J. L. & Horovitz, M. (2011). Parents' first concerns of their child's development in toddlers with autism spectrum disorders. *Developmental Neurorehabilitation.*, *14*, 72–78.

Kulesza, R. J., Jr. Lukose, R. & Stevens, L. V. (2011). Malformation of the human superior olive in autistic spectrum disorders. *Brain Res*, *1367*, 360-371.

Madell, J. R. (2014). Evaluation of hearing in children with special needs. In *Pediatric audiology*, (pp. 95-101). New York, NY: Thieme.

Manes, F., Piven, J., Vrancic, D., Nanclares, V., Plebst, C. & Starkstein, S. E. (1999). An MRI study of the corpus callosum and cerebellum in mentally retarded autistic individuals. *J. Neurophychiatry Clin Neurosci*, *11*, 470-474.

Meinzen-Derr, J., Wiley, S., Bishop, S., Manning- Courtney, P., Choo, D. & Murrary, D. (2014). Autism spectrum disorders in 24 children who are deaf or hard of hearing. *International Journal of Pediatric Otorhinolaryngology.*, *78*, 112-118.

Merzenich, M. M., Schreiner, C., Jenkins, W. & Wang, X. (1993). Neural mechanisms underlying temporal integration, segmentation, and input sequence representation: Some implications for the origin of learning disabilities. *Annals of the New York Academy of Sciences*, *682*, 1–21.

Mitchell, C., Phillips, D. S. & Trune, D. R. (1989). Variables affecting the auditory brainstem response: Audiogram, age, gender and head size. *Hearing Research*, *40*, 75–85.

Miron, O., Beam, A. L. & Kohane, I. S. (2018). Auditory Brainstem Response in Infants and Children with Autism Spectrum Disorder: A Meta-Analysis of Wave V. *Autism Research*, *11*, 355–363.

Musiek, F. E. & Pinheiro, M. L. (1985). Dichotic speech tests in the detection of central auditory dysfunction. In: Pinheiro, M. L. & Musiek, F. E. (Eds) *Assessment of Central Auditory Dysfunction: Foundations and Clinical Correlates*. Baltimore: Williams & Wilkins, pp. 201-217.

Prieve, B. A. & Stevens, F. (2000). The New York state universal newborn hearing screening demonstration projects: introduction and overview. *Ear Hear*, *21*, 85-91.

Recanzone, G. H., Schreiner, C. E. & Merzenich, M. M. (1993). Plasticity in the frequency representation of primary auditory cortex following discrimination training in adult owl monkeys. *J Neurosci.*, *13*, 87– 103.

Roper, L., Arnold, P. & Monteiro, B. (2003). Co-occurrence of autism and deafness: diagnostic considerations. *Autism*, *7*, 245-53.

Rosenhall, U., Nordin, V., Sandstrom, M., Ahlsen, G. & Gillberg, C. (1999). Autism and hearing loss. *Journal of Autism and Developmental Disorders*, *29*, 349-357.

Russo, Nicol T., Trommer, B., Zecker, S. & Kraus, N. (2009). Brainstem transcription of speech is disrupted in children with autism spectrum disorders. *Dev. Science*, *12*, 557–567. doi: 10.1111/j.1467-7687.2008.00790.x.

Schafer, E., Mathews, l., Smita, M., Hill, M., Munoz, A., Bishop, R. & Maloney, M. (2012). Personal FM systems for children with autism spectrum disorders (ASD) and/or attention-deficit hyperactivity disorder (ADHD): An initial investigation. *Journal of Communication Disorders*, *46*, 30–52.

Smith, D., Miller, S., Stewart, M., Walter, T. & McConnell, J. (1988). Conductive hearing loss in autistic, learning disabled and normal children. *J Autism Dev Dis*, *18*, 53–65 10.

Sugishita, M., Otomo, K., Yamazaki, K., Shimizu, H., Yoshioka, M. & Shinohara, A. (1995). Dichotic listening in patients with partial section of the corpus callosum. *Brain*, *118*, 417-427.

Szymanski, C., Brice, P., Lam, K. & Hotto, S. (2012). Deaf children with autism spectrum disorders. *Journal of Autism and Developmental Disorders*, *42*(10), 2027-2037.

Szymanski, A. & Johnston, J. (2018). Dually diagnosed autism and hearing loss. *The ASHA Leader*, 20-21.

Tharpe, A. M., Bess, F. H., Sladen, D. P., Schissel, H., Couch, S. & Schery, T. (2006). Auditory characteristics of children with autism. *Ear Hear*, *27*, 430 – 441.

Waiter, G. D., Williams, J. H., Murray, A. D., Gilchrist, A., Perrett, D. I. & Whiten, A. (2005). Structural white matter deficits in high functioning individuals with autistic spectrum disorder: A voxel-based investigation. *Neuroimage*, *24*, 455-461

Wilson, U. S., Sadler, K. M., Hancock, K. E., Guinan, J. J. Jr. & Lichtenhan, J. T. (2017). Efferent inhibition strength is a physiological correlate of hyperacusis in children with autism spectrum disorder. *Journal of Neurophysiology*, *118*, 1164-1172. DOI: 10.1152/ jn.00142.2017.

Wolff, J. J., Gu, H., Gerig, G., Elison, J. T., Styner, M., Gouttard, S. & Ibis Network. (2012). Differences in white matter fibertract development present from 6 to 24 months in infants with autism. *The American Journal of Psychiatry*, *169*, 589–600. doi: 10.1176/ appi.ajp .2011.11091447.

Worley, J. A., Matson, J. L. & Kozlowski, A. M. (2011). The effects of hearing impairment on symptoms of autism in toddler. *Developmental Neurorehabilitation*, *14*(3), 171-176.

In: Understanding Children with Autism … ISBN: 978-1-53617-647-6
Editor: Anne Bourque


*Chapter 3*

# DEVELOPMENTAL INTERVENTIONS FOR CHILDREN WITH AUTISM SPECTRUM DISORDERS: A LITERATURE REVIEW

***Magda Di Renzo[1], MD, Viviana Guerriero[1], PhD, Valeria Mammarella[2], MD and Federico Bianchi di Castelbianco[1], MD***

[1]Institute of Ortofonologia (IdO) of Rome, Rome, Italy
[2]Sapienza University of Rome, Rome, Italy

## ABSTRACT

Developmental approaches characterized interventions based on the typical sequences of the child's development, paying particular attention to the linguistic, motor and socio-emotional aspects, within a relational perspective. The purpose of this paper was to identify developmental interventions for children with Autism Spectrum Disorders (ASD) aged between 0 and 12 years old. A literature review was carried out searching on MEDLINE, PsycINFO, and PsycARTICLES and manually on key journals and reference lists of key articles. All the electronic databases have been consulted by setting a range of year of publication between 2009 and 2019, and only articles in English have been considered. Two reviewers assessed studies against predetermined inclusion criteria and 72 unique studies met our inclusion criteria. The interventions selected were described and the main outcomes discussed. This review highlights the need for improved research on intervention programs and the important service needs for families and children with Autism Spectrum Disorders.

**Keywords:** developmental interventions, autism spectrum disorder, children, psychotherapy

## INTRODUCTION

According to the Diagnostic and Statistical Manual of Mental Disorders (DSM-5) of the American Psychiatric Association [1] Autism Spectrum Disorders (ASD) are diagnosed in presence of persistent communication and social interaction deficits and restricted or repetitive interests or activities, emerging from the early stages of child development.

In recent years there has been an increase in the prevalence of Autism Spectrum Disorders. A 2012 systematic review [2] presenting epidemiological investigations since 2000 on ASD and Pervasive Developmental Disorders (PDD) worldwide, showed that the median of prevalence estimates was 12/10,000 children (range 2.8–94) and 62/10,000 children (range 1-189) respectively. A more recent review [3] showed a prevalence range of 21.7 cases (children and adolescents) every 10,000 in 24 countries. The studies found by these authors were then divided into those that were published from 1966 to 2000 (29 studies) and those that had been published from 2001 to 2013 (43 studies) and a prevalence of 11.9 cases every 10,000 and 28.4 cases per 10,000 respectively emerged, showing a significant increase in prevalence over the years. The authors also presented data supporting the hypothesis that DSM-5 diagnostic criteria for ASD applied to studies with samples diagnosed with DSM-IV [4] or DSM-IV-TR [5], did not facilitate the identification of individuals with ASD. The data presented in this study suggest what is also indicated by other authors [6], namely that the estimates prevalence for ASD may depend on several factors like the age range of the target population, the diagnostic manual, or the social system in which the investigation is conducted.

In a recent study [7], the prevalence of this disorder in 4 States (United States) among 4-year-olds individuals ranged from 13.4 per 1,000 children in 2012 to 17.0 per 1,000 children in 2014, while the prevalence of this disorder in 11 States among 8-year-olds individuals ranged from 13.1 to 29.3 per 1,000 children in 2014, with an m/f ratio of 4 to 1 [8]. This study also showed a comparison between the prevalence detected using the DSM-IV-TR and the DSM-5 for the diagnosis of ASD, and highlighted an overlapping of approximately 86% of cases, with a decrease in diagnosed cases using DSM-5.

European prevalence data from the 2018 network "Autism Spectrum Disorders in the European Union" (ASDEU) out of a total of 631,619 children recruited, found a prevalence of 12.2 children per 1,000 (1 in 89) aged 7 and 9 years, ranging from 4.4 to 19.7 children per 1,000 [9].

For a more comprehensive view of the Italian context, we report below some of the most recent prevalence studies. According to ISTAT data published in 2018 on the position of students with disabilities in primary and secondary schools, for the school year 2016-2017, 25.6% of pupils with disabilities in primary school and 21.7% of pupils with disabilities in lower secondary school have been diagnosed with a developmental disorders (Autism Spectrum Disorders) with a prevalence of 0.84% of the total [10]. A recent study that aimed to assess the prevalence of ASD in 10,138 children aged 7 to 9 in the province of Pisa (Italy) estimated a 0.79% prevalence [11]. Finally, data from two Italian regions (Piemonte and Emilia Romagna) indicate a prevalence of PDD in the 6-10 age group of 4.2/1000 children in 2010 and 2.8/1000 children in 2011 [6]. The serious data of ASD prevalence and the high complexity of this disorder demand for deepening the study of interventions aimed at children with ASD.

## DEVELOPMENTAL THERAPIES FOR CHILDREN WITH AUTISM SPECTRUM DISORDER

Despite the high importance of early and appropriate interventions addressing children's and families' needs to promote positive outcomes, considerable variation regarding both access to interventions and the type of intervention received emerges across countries [12].

A study involving 1,680 parents of children with ASD from 18 European countries (Belgium, Czech Republic, Denmark, Finland, France, Germany, Hungary, Iceland, Ireland, Italy, The Netherlands, Norway, Poland, Portugal, Romania, Spain, the former Yugoslav Republic of Macedonia and the United Kingdom), aimed at collecting data about the interventions provided to children aged 7 and under. Data showed that 91% used at least one type of intervention among behavioral intervention, developmental and/or relationship-based intervention, speech and language therapy, occupational therapy, other educational and psychological interventions or parent training [12]. The speech and language therapies were the most widely used, while the behavioral, developmental and/or relationship-based interventions accounted for 45% among those applied, representing the second most widely used type of intervention in all the countries involved. Furthermore, the developmental and relationship-based therapies were most commonly used in southern and eastern Europe.

In this field, we can identify several developmental interventions, but among them we can find some core characteristics that seem useful to clarify [13]. The first key feature concerns the strong link with the scientific theories and knowledge of the developmental approach, which also include Attachment Theory and Infant Research [14, 15, 16, 17, 18, 19]. Developmental theories guide both assessment and intervention planning. These interventions consider the importance of critical period (or developmental windows) in common to all children for the promotion and the acquisition of essential skills. Simultaneously they consider the importance to set specific goals for each individual, bearing in mind both risk and protective factors [20]. Great importance is also given to the child's relationship with significant adults and reciprocal social interactions [21]. In this perspective, the child is seen as an active subject who participates, interacts and co-constructs the therapy [22]. Finally, developmental approaches typically use play sessions to encourage spontaneity, initiative, motivations and provides them opportunities to engage in interpersonal relationships [23, 24, 25]. In sum, developmental approaches characterized interventions based on the typical sequences of the child's development, paying particular attention to the linguistic, motor and socio-emotional aspects, within a relational perspective.

Before proceeding with our review, it is necessary to give a short mention of early intervention for toddler-aged children (from birth to 36 months) with or at risk of ASD. The identification of ASD in toddler-aged children has begun especially important in the past decade, to identify positive prognostic indicators and to plan adequate psycho-educational interventions to support the child's development [26]. A 2011 review [27] identified 14 different developmental domains among 27 papers selected: joint attention, motivation, acceptable behavior or compliance, communication, play, imitation, turn-taking, social interaction, eye contact or looking at faces, cognition, adaptive/self-help, motor, sensory and affect/social-emotional. The majority of the interventions focused on joint attention or communication areas. Among these early interventions, the majority were conducted out of the natural child environment and by professionals as the principal agents of intervention, rather than parents. Furthermore, this paper stated that less than half interventions reviewed promote internal child motivation or child initiative in learning and that all the interventions reported using functional systematic intervention methods "not always easily determined from descriptions provided" (p. 17) [27]. About developmentally targeted interventions, the authors concluded that they varied in their accounting of the role of developmental foundations in their work, especially for the social communication area, and that additional study is needed for distinguishing developmental outcomes of interventions targeting joint attention and those aimed at more developmentally remote abilities.

## METHODS OF THE LITERATURE REVIEW

The survey methodology for the current literature review was based on the use of Medline, PsycArticles, PsycInfo, ProQuest and Psychology electronic database, using the following combination of keywords: "autism" or "ASD" or "Autism Spectrum Disorder" and "developmental intervention" or "developmental treatment" or "developmental therapy". All electronic databases were consulted in a publication range between 2009 and 2019, considering studies carried out on the population of children aged from 0 to 12 years. Only full-text articles in English were considered, and all papers other than journal articles or book chapters, including book reviews, commentaries, and dissertations, were excluded. Additional scientific articles were found by manually examining key scientific journals in this area and references of key articles. Finally, 72 scientific articles dealing with the topic of interest of this review have been selected.

## THE DEVELOPMENTAL INDIVIDUAL-DIFFERENCES, RELATIONSHIP-BASED MODEL

The Developmental Individual-Differences, Relationship-Based Model (DIR®) was developed by Stanley Greenspan and Serena Weider [28] for understanding and promoting the positive development of children, focusing on a variety of children capacities. Greenspan has listed six steps or stages of typical development and the corresponding pathologies that might occur if a stage did not progress appropriately: the first stage is called "homeostasis" and it relates to the child internal regulation and a well-balanced interest in the world; the second stage is "attachment" and it is characterized by an emotional investment in animated world, especially caregivers; the third stage is about the "somatopsychological differentiation", typified by the child acquisition to be flexible, multisystem, affective within reciprocal interactions with primary caregivers; the fourth step concerns the child "behavioral organization, initiative, and internalization" in which the child creates more stable and organized mental representations that organize his/her behavior; the fifth stage, that is the "representational capacity, differentiation, and consolidation", is characterized by the consolidation of the child internal representations, the ability to evoke internal object and to organize multisensory experiences, resulting also in a stabilization of mood; the sixth stage occours from middle childhood through adolescence, and it is characterized by a gradual consolidation of derivative and multiple reppresentational systems, greater flexibility and ability to organize, integrate and differentiate a great amount of affective and ideational content. The failure in the development of adaptive capacities, usually matched by maladaptive caregiver behaviors, may conclude with regulatory disorders; autistic patterns; narrow, rigid or stereotyped responses to others, and random or chaotic behavior and affect; disorganized withdrawn, compliant, or aggressive behavior, stereotyped and polarized behavior and emotion; poor sense of self and others, concreteness of behavior and affect; impulse regulation, mood stabilization and compromised reality testing, depending on the developmental stage impaired. The typical outcomes described for each step represent core therapeutic goals in the treatment of children who have not acquired the abilities of a particular step.

DIRFloortime® (Floortime) is the application of the DIR model in a comprehensive intervention, commonly utilized with children with ASD or other developmental or socio-emotional challenges. It aims at working with the child on the abilities missed in his/her developmental process, through one-to-one interactions between a therapist and a trained parent. In order to accomplish this, the therapy is designed to stimulate child interest through play in a natural environment.

Pajareya and Nopmaneejumruslers [29] presented positive data confirming the results obtained by a previous pilot study [30] using the (DIR)/Floortime™ intervention for preschool children with ASD. Mercer [31] wrote an interesting review on theory and research of DIR/Floortime™ as a treatment for children with ASD, listing several adjuvant treatments to DIR/Floortime that seems to be less plausible. They include speech therapy [32], sensory integration theory (SIT) [33] and developmental optometry

[34]. Against this background, Au and Coulter [35] suggested combining traditional Vision Therapy (VT) techniques with the DIRFloortime model for providing a more comprehensive intervention for children with ASD. This paper also suggested that DIR/Floortime™ is congruent with the developmental theory about ASD, but it does not have the status of an evidence-based treatment yet, letting us deduce that additional randomized control trials are needed.

## THE JOINT ATTENTION, SYMBOLIC PLAY, ENGAGEMENT AND REGULATION

The Joint Attention, Symbolic Play, Engagement & Regulation (JASPER) [36] approach was developed by Connie Kasari with the goal of interacting with children with autism through naturalistic strategies to target the foundations of social-communication in terms of joint attention, imitation, and play. JASPER model is based on the assumption that joint attention and play skills represent a key component of the child's future ability of understanding other's mental representations, and as a consequence, they may positively influence children's social, cognitive, and language abilities [37]. On the basis of this model, a combined developmental and behavioral intervention was implemented, to improve joint attention and symbolic play skills in children with ASD, that are supposed to be characterized by significant deficits in social communication skills. This evidence-based social communication approach consists of approximately 3–6 months of service (minimum 24 sessions) conducted by clinicians, special education teachers or caregivers, typically delivered one-to-one, as well as in group/classroom sessions.

When 16 children were randomly assigned to 6-week JASPER intervention implemented by public school teachers or a control group, data showed more JASPER strategies used by teachers and more joint attention and more time in supported engagement in children of the JASPER group than the control group [36]. In a pilot study [38] the effects of JASPER were tested on a sample of 15 minimally verbal children with autism aged between 3 and 5 years old. Children were randomly assigned to the control group or JASPER intervention (implemented by graduate students in educational psychology). Data showed greater play diversity, more gestures and less time spent unengaged for children in JASPER treatment compared with the control group.

The JASPER intervention conducted by a caregiver was evaluated comparing children's improvements after a group of 24 sessions with 1year follow-up to control group of children in the waitlist and showing significant differences in targeted areas of joint engagement [39]. The intervention conducted by the caregiver was also evaluated in a study [40] comparing two small group training for caregivers with or without the child being present. Data showed that both intervention groups improved child outcome, but the caregiver group with the child being present was more effective when compared to the group without the child.

One study [41] compared a 10 weeks caregiver-child JASPER with a parent-only psychoeducational intervention, showing a significant effect of JASPER in dyadic joint engagement, and a significant effect of the parent-only psychoeducational intervention in reducing parenting stress associated with child characteristics.

Regarding teacher implementation, a 2016 study [42] highlighted that teachers and teaching assistants can deliver JASPER with high fidelity in their preschool classroom day, after a brief but sustained coaching support throughout the 2 months of intervention. Furthermore, significant effects in joint attention gestures, child-initiated joint engagement, joint attention language, and length of language emerged for children who have received 2 months of daily classroom JASPER, when compared to children in the waitlist. Shire and colleagues [43] also compared data on JASPER intervention or treatment on children with ASD living in low resource neighborhoods. Children were randomized to Joint Attention, Symbolic Play, Engagement, and Regulation or waitlist and results showed that teaching assistants implementation of JASPER intervention had an adequate fidelity and that children treated with JASPER had significant gains in joint engagement, joint attention, and play skills when compared to children in the waitlist. A more recent study [44] explored the fidelity of teacher assistants delivering JASPER, showing maintained quality implementation of many of the intervention strategies investigated. Data also showed that teaching assistants helped the children to get into longer periods of joint engagement and to maintain that level of engagement, during the second year of working.

One paper [45] expanded the results that emerged from the study by Almirall and colleagues [46], comparing the longitudinal improvement of minimally verbal children with a diagnosis of autism, aged between 5 and 8 years old. Two treatment (only JASPER and Enhanced Milieu Teaching intervention versus JASPER, Enhanced Milieu Teaching intervention and the use of a speech-generating device) outcomes were compared showing similar play level improvements over a 6-month intervention, but few differences between the two treatments.

According to this study's presentation, we can conclude that the data available on the efficacy of the JASPER approach in improving children's joint attention, and symbolic play skills were generally successfully achieved by different operators, but these results need to be replicated with larger sample size.

## The Early Start Denver Model Intervention

The Early Start Denver Model is a comprehensive developmental behavioral intervention for improving outcomes of infants to preschool-aged children with ASD. This intervention integrates Applied Behavior Analysis (ABA) with relationship-based and developmental theories, and it is provided in the children'snatural environment and delivered by trained therapists and parents.

Reports from the first studies using the ESDM delivered by therapists showed children decreasing of symptoms severity and improvements in children's development, especially in the language domain [47, 48, 49]. Children's improvements after this intervention were also associated with normalized patterns of brain activity when this intervention was compared with a community intervention [50]. A longitudinal study on 39 6-year-old children with ASD showed also that the gains were maintained and an improvement in core autism symptoms and adaptive behavior when compared with the group of intervention, as usual, two years after the intervention ended [51]. Rogers and colleagues [52] replicated and extended the 2010 study by Dawson and colleagues [47], in which the outcomes of forty-eight children diagnosed with ASD between 18 and 30 months of age were compared when assigned to an ESDM intervention or an intervention as usual, demonstrating the efficacy of this developmental behavioral intervention for toddlers with ASD.

A 2016 review [53] indicated positive child, parent, and therapist outcomes reported in the identified studies, but it also showed a weakness in terms of effectiveness. Recently one study [54] on a parent-implemented Early Start Denver Model (P-ESDM) was implemented with one hundred eighteen children aged between 14 to 24 months and parents to determine its efficacy for children outcomes. A short-term intervention for toddlers with ASD lasting twelve weeks was compared with an enhanced ESDM version, including also motivational interviewing, multimodal learning tools, and a weekly home visit. Parents in the enhanced ESDM group showed increased sensitivity and skills in supporting children's development as compared to the parents of the control group, while children showed similar gains for both groups over time.

Further implementation of ESDM is based on the delivery of this intervention in group-based settings. In this context, a recent review [55] described it as a feasible and sustainable early intervention for young autistic children, that is showing initial promising data. This data was confirmed by a 2019 study involving 44 preschoolers children with ASD receiving the Group-Early Start Denver Model in classroom setting [56], in which children showed improvements and mothers experienced a reduction in stress. Nevertheless, this review stressed the importance of deepening the community viability of this model, the permanence of activities and resources after the training, and the long-term outcomes.

## Milieu Teaching

The Milieu Teaching (MT) [57] is an intervention for children focused on teaching new communication skills and behaviors within children's natural settings (i.e., home or school). It was performed with children with ASD and is about modeling children's correct responses and correcting them as necessary. It includes a social interactionist perspective, with an emphasis on parents as interventionists [58]. There are several versions of the Milieu Teaching approach including Milieu Language Teaching (MT) [59], Milieu Communication Teaching (MCT) [60] and Prelinguistic Milieu Teaching (PMT) [61], taking into account additional environmental variables to that of the traditional Milieu Teaching.

Christensen-Sandfort and Whinnery [62] examined the effectiveness of the Milieu Teaching classroom intervention for young children during a period of 5 months. Participants attended a preschool classroom for children with varying exceptionalities, and the intervention was provided by a trained teacher. This paper demonstrated the positive impact of the Milieu strategies in increasing spontaneous speech in children with ASD and the usefulness of this intervention for teachers of young children with ASD during classroom activities.

The Prelinguistic Milieu Teaching (PMT) [61] targets prelinguistic social communication outcomes (i.e., eye gaze, gestures, vocalizations) used to request and share attention and it is embedded in play routines within a child's natural environment. Six non-verbal children aged between 5 and 8 years old, with a diagnosis of autism were taught to initiate communication using vocalizations, gestures, and eye gaze within play routines. Data revealed an improvement in children's number of communicative interactions during play routines and initiated intentional communication [58]. One recent paper [63] has deepened the efficacy and the feasibility of PMT with three preschoolers with or at risk for ASD in the context of their classrooms, showing an increase in their engagement in communicative acts.

Another implementation of this intervention is the Responsivity Education/Prelinguistic Milieu Teaching (RE/PMT) therapy consisting of both Prelinguistic Milieu Teaching delivered to the children and responsivity education delivered to the parents. The Responsivity Education deals with teaching parents to be highly responsive to their children's intentional and unintentional communication and focus of attention, waiting for their child to initiate vocal/motor behaviors and providing proper behaviors as a consequence of their child communication [64]. Yoder and Lieberman [65] compared thirty-six children outcomes comparing RE/PMT or Picture Exchange Communication System (PECS) sessions per week for 6 months and revealed that children receiving RE/PMT intervention were lower in the picture exchanges compared to children receiving in a generalized context. Mcduffie and colleagues [66] compared thirty-two children with ASD aged 18–60 months outcomes when randomly assigned to the (PECS) or RE/PMT treatments. This paper showed that object interest in young children with ASD in the RE/PMT intervention showed a gain in object interest as compared to children in the PECS intervention.

The Enhanced Milieu Teaching (EMT) [59] is an evidence-based and manualized language intervention based on "a naturalistic model of early language intervention in which child interest and initiations are used as opportunities to model and prompt language use in everyday contexts" (p. 296) [67]. It is delivered by a parent and therapist or only by a therapist, who uses developmentally responsive strategies and behavioral teaching strategies to improve children's language. The study by Kaiser and Roberts [67] showed more gains in preschool children receiving EMT implemented by parents and therapist when compared with the control group of therapist-only EMT. When Jasper plus EMT intervention with or without the augmentation of a speech-generating device (SGD) was provided to sixty-one children with autism, aged 5 to 8 years, received a JASP+EMT intervention, data showed that a JASP+EMT intervention incorporating an SGD had a significant and rapid gain in children language [68]. A recent study [69] deepened the effects of the EMT implemented by the therapist on three children with ASD in South Africa and highlighted an increase in the number of words and the number of spontaneous utterances expressed by the children.

In sum, as revealed in a 2009 review on early research conducted in the area of Milieu Therapy, this intervention revealed an increase in children targeted communication skills [69], while a more recent review [71] suggested a lack of consistency and the need of better define the quality and the quantity of these interventions. Studies investigating Milieu interventions are also limited in terms of participants' age, diagnosis, language severity, and intellectual functioning, and these aspects should be further explored.

## Treatment and Education of Autistic and Related Communication Handicapped Children

The Treatment and Education of Autistic and Related Communication Handicapped Children (TEACCH) [72] is a comprehensive treatment method using children preferred activities that are supposed to be more easy to understand, practice, and generalize. The primary aim of this intervention is to improve many different areas of an individual's development, focusing on children's strengths, interests, and needs [73]. This treatment relies on traditional behavioral, neo-behavioral and developmental techniques, usually as part of classroom-based programs of structured teaching. Within this model, the Structured Teaching is a set of teaching principles and intervention strategies helping practictioners' understanding of children needs and learning styles [74]. Children are supported in processing information visually and in choosing, engaging in, and making sense of daily activities. Parents are trained as co-therapists, so home-based programs are also possible. TEACCH programs are not based on children typical development and do not include a standardized curriculum for each child, but they pay attention to the following key elements: "organization of the physical environment, visual information, task organization, and work systems" (pag. 429) [75]. The development of this treatment relies on Eric Schopler theories hypothesizing a better chance for children with autism to learn through visual perceptions than through auditory perceptions, and to have better outcomes when the interventions take place in structured sessions than in unstructured sessions [76]. A 2013 meta-analysis [77] of intervention studies[1] about TEACCH program for children and adults with autism provided limited support for the clinical effects of the TEACCH program (see Table 1). But nevertheless, Virues-Ortega and colleagues [75] underline that the 2013 review shows also evidence for good practice in TEACCH program like the standardized assessments, the presence of semi-independent international teams, and training carried directly by the first TEACCH center. Besides, reviewed studies in 2013 showed better gains in adaptive, verbal, cognitive, perceptual and motor areas among older participants (6–17 years of age) then younger children (0–5 years of age).

Some authors [78] compared ABA and TEACCH treatment models applied at students with ASD, also studying their comprehensiveness and fidelity, concluding that there is no reliable data for favoring one approach over the other; that parents, teachers, and administrators did not prefer one intervention over the other; but they rated as significantly valid some components specific to autism treatment of both approaches. The outcome of TEACCH treatment was also compared to that of children on the waiting list. A pilot randomized controlled trial [79] recruited eleven children with High Functioning Autism, aged between 5 and 6 years old and their mothers, showing better improvements if the individuals were assigned to the TEACCH program than to the control group. When the TEACCH was compared to the LEAP (Learning Experiences - An Alternative Program for Preschoolers and Parents) intervention. A study from our review shows that teachers in special education programs showed a similar level of commitment to both programs in teachers [80] and children [81], although for TEACCH more beneficial to children with greater cognitive impairments emerged.

---

[1] The papers published since 2009 and cited in this meta-analysis [77] were considered in our review but not extensively descripted.

**Table 1. List of papers included in the Virues-Ortega, Julio and Pastor (2013) meta-analysis**

| Papers | Participants age (years) |
|---|---|
| Aoyama, S. (1995). "The efficacy of structuring the work system: Individualization of the work format and the use of a 3-level paper rack in a special education class." [82] | School age |
| Ozonoff, S., & Cathcart, K. (1998). "Effectiveness of a home program intervention for young children with autism." [83] | 4,4 |
| Persson, B. (2000). "Brief report: A longitudinal study of quality of life and independence among adult men with autism." [84] | 32,3 |
| Panerai, S., Ferrante, L., & Zingale, M. (2002). "Benefits of the Treatment and Education of Autistic and Communication Handicapped Children (TEACCH) programme as compared with a non-specific approach." [85] | 9,1 |
| Van Bourgondien, M. E., Reichle, N. C., & Schopler, E. (2003). "Effects of a model treatment approach on adults with autism." [86] | 23,7 |
| Siaperas, P., & Beadle-Brown, J. (2006). "A case study of the use of a structured teaching approach in adults with autism in a residential home in Greece." [87] | 21,3 |
| Siaperas, P., Higgins, S., & Proios, P. (2007). "Challenging behaviors on people with autism: A case study on the effect of a residential training programme based on structured teaching and TEACCH method." [88] | 21,3 |
| Tsang, S., Shek, D., Lam, L., Tang, F., & Cheung, P. (2007). "Brief report: Application of the TEACCH program on Chinese pre-school children with autism — Does culture make a difference?" [89] | 4,6 years |
| Probst, P., & Leppert, T. (2008). "Brief report: Outcomes of a teacher training program for autism spectrum disorders." [90] | 10,0 years |
| Panerai, S., Zingale, M., Trubia, G., Finocchiaro, M., Zuccarello, R., Ferrei, R., et al. (2009). "Special education versus inclusive education: The TEACCH program." [91] | 8,7 years<br>9,7 years |
| McConkey, R., Truesdale-Kennedy, M., Crawford, H., McGreevy, E., Reavey, M., & Cassidy, A. (2010). "Preschoolers with autism spectrum disorders: Evaluating the impact of a home-based intervention to promote their communication." [92] | 2,8 |

| Papers | Participants age (years) |
|---|---|
| Braiden, H. J., McDaniel, B., McCrudden, E., Hanes, M., & Crozier, B. (2012). "A practice-based evaluation of Barnardo's forward steps early intervention programme for children diagnosed with autism." [93] | 3,2 |
| Welterlin, A., Turner-Brown, L. M., Harris, S., Mesibov, G., & Delmolino, L. (2012). "The home TEACCHing program for toddlers with autism." [94] | 2,5 |

Note. The black line distinguishes the papers published before and after 2009.
R-TEACCH= residential TEACCH; NS-TEACCH= natural setting TEACCH.

An implementation of the TEACCH is the Family Implemented TEACCH for Toddlers (FITT), designed for improving the services intended to occur in children's natural settings like homes (usually called Part C). This parent-mediated approach aims at enhancing parental skills for better targeting the needs, understanding and engaging with toddlers with ASD. In a 2016 study [95] forty-nine participants were recruited and randomly assigned to FITT or services as usual. For FITT intervention approach positive effects on parents' stress and their mental well-being, no specific treatment effect on children's developmental skills, and better toddler social communication outcomes emerged.

In conclusion, this review of studies about the TEACCH highlights that this intervention model incorporates techniques from different perspectives, that more evidence of effectiveness is needed, and key concepts of the intervention are not fully operationalized [75].

## HANEN'S 'MORE THAN WORDS'

Hanen's 'More than Words' (HMTW) [96] is a parent-implemented training program targeted in enhancing children's communication/language and consisting of eight weekly group sessions and three individual family sessions. The HMTW program consists of enhancing parents' responsivity to children's attention and communication signals, increasing the frequency of playful parent–child interactions and facilitate children's communication, through support, education, and practical skills.

Parents are taught to structure everyday routines with the aim of improving parent–child interactions in a more sensitive way, providing more appropriate verbal and non-verbal stimuli to children's communication [97].

Since 2009 there are only few studies investigating HMTW, to our knowledge. One pilot study [98] recruited four families of children with ASD aged between 37 months to 69 months pointing out that HMTW had a positive impact on children's social interaction and vocabulary development. The study by Carter and colleagues [96] enrolled 62 children aged 15–25 months with autism and their parents. Children were assigned to either the experimental treatment or to a community treatment but no significant differences between the two interventions were found on parental responsivity and children's communication. In contrast, there were improvements in communication depending on children's levels of object interest at the beginning of treatment, showing that this intervention had better effects on child communication with early lower levels of object interest. Fifty children with ASD, and aged 1- 5 years were recruited in a 2017 study [99] to explore the effectiveness of the HMTW intervention programfor ASD children. This study showed significant improvements in children's level of communication and activities, including joint attention, turntaking, eye contact, and toilet training, over time.

Finally, in 2018 a study [100] about the effectiveness of HMTW on parents of children with ASD in Malaysia was conducted. Thirty-one children with ASD and their parents were recruited and assigned either to intervention or control group. Data showed a significant increase in responsive interactions, the retention of facilitative strategies in parents during time, and higher levels of satisfaction than parents in the control group.

As shown above, data on the effectiveness of the HMTW treatment are promising, but further studies are needed to support the use of this intervention.

## Preschool Autism Communication Trial

The Preschool Autism Communication Trial (PACT) [101] is a parent-child communication-focused intervention for children with core autism, aged between 2 and 5 years. This treatment targets "increasing parental sensitivity to child communication and reducing mistimed responses using video feedback, and [...] promoting a range of positive social communication strategies" [102] (page. 427). According to this approach the intervention consists of sessions between therapist and parents with the child present, with the aim of increasing parental sensitivity and responsiveness to child communication, and the help of video-feedback methods to address parent-child interaction.

A first study [101] exploring this kind of intervention compared children's gains when randomly assigned to PACT or intervention as usual. Data demonstrated an improvement in both groups, with a little difference in favor of the PACT intervention, and better perceptions of children's language and social communication by parents of the PACT group. A 2015 paper [103] explored the direct and indirect effects of PACT on child behavior and ADOS-G score via parent behavior. Data suggested the mediating role of the parent synchrony and child initiations on the ADOS-G score and supported the PACT theoretical model.

In a subsequent follow-up of this study [104], it was found a reduction of autism symptoms in both autism repetitive symptom and social-communication domains, until 6 years later the treatment endpoint. Similar results to the 2010 study were found in a research [105] conducted in south Asia, India and Pakistan for 64 children aged 2–9 years. A more recent study [106] recruited a sample of caregivers of children with autism aged 8–12 years and did not find a specific protective effect of PACT on parenting stress and well-being, over and above the effect of all the other risk factors.

The results of these studies are not fully promising at present, though more research on the effectiveness of this intervention is needed.

## JOINT ATTENTION MEDIATED LEARNING

The Joint Attention Mediated Learning (JAML) [107] is a recent parent-mediated interaction-based intervention for toddlers with ASD, focused on children's social functions of preverbal communication. This intervention is driven by 5 main concepts adapted by Klein's [108] principles of mediated learning: parents should help their children focusing their attention on the objectives, organizing and planning to communicate socially (improving self-regulation), encouraging self-confidence, giving meaning of socially important interaction cues, and expanding interactions in varied settings and with different people.

The JAML includes three phases targeted on the acquisition of joint attention and other early social communication abilities. During the first phase (Focusing on Faces, FF), the child is aided in looking to the parent's face, during the second phase (Turn-Taking, TT) the child is helped in engaging with the parent in play interactions; during the third phase (Joint Attention, JA) the child is engaged in triadic interactions using toys. The authors also stressed that the focus of this intervention is on social rather than instrumental communicative functions [109].

A 2013 study [107] aimed at examining the efficacy of JAML for promoting joint attention and early communication for toddlers with ASD. Twenty-three parents and their children were recruited and were randomly assigned to JAML intervention or a control condition. Data showed more frequent responses to parents' joint attention approaches and improvement in children's communication, guiding children learning from simpler to more complex forms of preverbal social communication. Another study [110] recruited 144 children with ASD aged 16–30 months and their parents to examine the efficacy and implementation of the JAML intervention in promoting children's early social communication. The children were randomly assigned to JAML or community control conditions. Results showed sustaining treatment differences over 6 months after intervention, nevertheless to our knowledge there are still few studies investigating the effectiveness of the JAML intervention.

## THE DEVELOPMENTAL, EMOTIONAL REGULATION, RELATIONSHIP AND BODY-BASED INTERVENTION

The Developmental, Emotional regulation, Relationship and Body-Based model (DERBBI) [111] is an approach that attaches great importance to the connection between affect, motor planning and sequencing (see the "affective diathesis" by Greenspan [112]), in the core deficit of children with ASD. Within this model was developed a specific intervention for children with ASD: the Turtle Project. The Turtle Project [113] is an individualized intervention based on an individual's profile to use developmentally appropriate and meaningful targets. This profile is developed thanks to an accurate diagnostic process, including the TULIP protocol [114], for a comprehensive assessment of the predictors of positive outcomes in children with ASD.

In this model, the diagnostic process is carried out by a group of experts (psychologists, neuropsychiatrists, and other specialized figures) with the means to select targets and measures according to the specific child, useful for early indicators of treatment and follow-up monitoring.

The Turtle Project generally plans to improve parent-child affective attunement, the child-peer imitation process, and the child's ability to integrate and process sensory perceptions, during the first year of therapy. The second year of intervention typically refers to the psychomotor/ communicative-relational area, with the aim of improving children's motor initiative and emotion regulation, towards the re-definition of their body schema. During the third year, this intervention commonly aims to improve children's linguistic, behavioral, relational, cognitive, playing skills, personal autonomy and motivation to relate with. Finally, during the fourth year the intervention keeps improving the children verbal and non-verbal relational strategies, with a focus on the school learning. At this stage a special attention is paid to the holophony technique. This is a sound reproduction technique that simulates human listening strategies by immersing the listener in a three-dimensional hearing reality. Through sound-motor and graphic-interactive paths and games children are driven to improve emotion regulation, visual-spatial, speech, and learning abilities and executive functioning [115].

The targets of the Turtle Project are met through the combination of different settings: group settings for children with similar functioning levels, parent-child dyadic and triadic settings, parents support groups, school support service and animal-assisted therapy. The treatment has an average duration of 4 years and it consists of 10 hours of treatment per week including 6 hours of child individual/group therapy, 2 hours of parental support, and 2 hours of school observation and counseling [111].

The Turtle Project is an example of a program that both reflects and contributes to the evidence base of autism interventions, through various studies that have shown an assessment protocol useful for capturing the complexity and the uniqueness of every child [114, 116, 117]. Furthermore, the studies deepening the effectiveness of the Turtle Project highlighted the protective factors identified during the diagnostic assessment and useful in predicting children's developmental trajectories and children for whom this type of treatment could lead to a greater improvement in symptoms [113, 114, 118, 119]. Third, recent papers have brought new reflections on the need to customize the intervention according to the characteristics not only of the autistic disorder but above all of the child and his/her family.

More specifically, in the 2015 paper [118] on a sample of 90 individuals with ASD aged between 2 years and six months and 16 years, data showed an improvement in autistic symptoms after 4 years of treatment. The 2016 paper [113] provided further data supporting the effectiveness of Turtle Project, indicating that after two and four years of treatment children exhibited a significant improvement in all assessed areas (speech and communication, mutual social interaction, play, restricted and repetitive behaviors, and Intelligence Quotient), in addition to a significant reduction in core autistic symptoms.

In this context, research studies should try to identify a specific population among the autisms, that could get better improvements from this type of developmental intervention, that gives special emphasis to the body and relational aspects.

## IMPROVING PARENTS AS COMMUNICATION TEACHERS (PROJECT IMPACT)

The Improving Parents As Communication Teachers Project (ImPACT) is a training for parents' intervention to promote children's social engagement, language, social imitation, and play during daily routines [120]. It can be implemented in either a group or individual settings to teach parents first to promote their responsiveness and social reciprocity trough videotaped examples, homework written and spoken descriptions of techniques, and practice with coaching.

In a single-subject study [121], 8 children with their mothers were recruited to examine the efficacy of this model and showed an increase in parents' intervention techniques, children use of language, and a significant association between parents' abilities and children language. In 2015 a pilot study [122] compared ImPACT intervention group with the community group addressed to 30 children with ASD. The paper had the aim to explore the effectiveness of this intervention and showed a strong parent intervention adherence and a significant improvement in the child's social-communication skills.

The Project ImPACT for Toddlers is a toddler-specific adaptation of ImPACT that included a parent-mediated intervention specifically addressed to 12 to 36 months children, and focused on improving children's play, social engagement, communication, and imitation in children's natural setting. It provides to parents brief didactic information sessions alternate with practice sessions with clinician feedback [123]. Recently, some authors [124] compared parent-child improvements when children where assigned to either the Project ImPACT for Toddlers or usual care and showed more positive parent–child interactions and children's social and communication skills, for individuals in the Project ImPACT for Toddlers group than usual care group.

Limited data from clinical studies support the effectiveness of this intervention, that however needs further monitoring and investigations.

## FURTHER DEVELOPMENTAL INTERVENTIONS

This section aims to mention recently or poorly investigated developmental interventions for children with ASD, as revealed by our literature review.

As part of intervention focused on joint attention, a recent study [118] described a brief parent-mediated home-based intervention focused on joint attention, imitation and social engagement skills of children with ASD. This study compared improvements in children and parents who underwent this specific intervention or a intervention as usual, over five sessions. Data showed significant improvements in children and lower levels of perceived stress and better coping in parents of the parent-mediated intervention group when compared to parents of the intervention as usual, along with high fidelity of intervention and parental adherence to the parent-mediated intervention.

In the broader framework of early intervention programs for children with autism, data suggest the positive effects of interventions focused on joint attention and play skills, with a lack or limited follow-up data. In this context, one long-term follow-up study by Kasari and colleagues [126] recruited a sample of children with autism assigned to joint attention (JA), symbolic play (SP), or control (CO) group. Results showed that a comprehensive intervention targeting joint attention and play skills positively affects the children long-term language outcomes.

As part of the parent-mediated interventions, we mention the *Pathways Early Autism Intervention* [127, 128]. It is a community-based, intensive behavioral and developmental intervention program for toddlers with ASD. According to this intervention, parent-child interactions are video recorded and reviewed with the parent, providing feedback on intervention strategies. The interventionist introduces new topics, clarifies parent questions, demonstrates new strategies with the child, plans activities and routines. This intervention is aimed to promote children's communication and social engagement. In a pilot study [126] for demonstrating its effectiveness, four boys with ASD and their mothers were recruited and the authors found that this intervention program is useful for improving children's early social communication but not for nonverbal turn-taking. Furthermore, a 2019 study [129] stressed that parents in the Pathways group experienced a decrease in stress levels and an increase in responsiveness when compared with parents in the control group.

The *Relationship Development Intervention* (RDI) [130, 131] is a parent-delivered intervention aimed at improving children's emotional referencing, declarative language, social coordination, relational information processing, flexible thinking, and foresight and hindsight of children with ASD. The intervention is implemented by parents who learn to perceive and support their children's perceptual, cognitive, and emotional patterns through a intensive training in RDI theory, principles, and components. A modified version of the RDI was recently implemented in China [132]. Forty-two children were recruited and assigned to RDI or a control group. Results showed better improvements in language, social, sensory and behavioral domains than those in the control group, after a 6 months training.

The *Responsive Teaching* (RT) [133], is a parent-mediated developmental intervention focused on children's communication, cognition, and social-emotional domains. Parents are trained to address their children with responsive interaction strategies to reach 19 predefined objectives within daily routines. Data on RT intervention shows an improvement in children developmental and social-emotional functioning and parents' responsiveness and affect [134, 135]. In a recent study [136], a sample of 28 Saudi Arabian children and their parents were recruited, and mothers who participated in Responsive Teaching intervention showed improvements in parenting stress and depression.

The *Video-feedback Intervention to promote Positive Parenting adapted to Autism* (VIPP-AUTI) is a video feedback attachment-based intervention program, aiming to enhance parental sensitivity to their child's signals and improving parent–child interaction [137]. This is an adapted version of the original VIPP by Juffer and colleagues [138], already employed in various families of infants, toddlers and preschoolers. The VIPP-AUTI program comprise a short-term parent-child interaction, videotaped in a natural environment, with video feedback. Data showed [139] a decrease in parental intrusiveness towards the child and an increase in parental efficacy. Significant differences between VIPP-AUTI and control group emerged in child-initiated joint attention skills, at follow-up.

Finally, among the studies reviewed as part of the play intervention, we found the *Play and Language for Autistic Youngsters* (PLAY) [140] model that is a parent-mediated developmental model focused on helping parents to increase their interaction with the child, and children to improve their social interaction and emotional development. This intervention is shown to be effective in parental responsiveness, affect and depression and children's social engagement [140, 141].

## CONCLUSION

As stated by Zhou and colleagues [49] the Naturalistic Developmental Behavioral Interventions (NDBIs) "integrate developmental and relationship-based approaches with strategies of applied behavior analysis, and emphasize establishing joint activity routines in natural environments, including play and daily life activities in which many learning opportunities can be embedded" (p. 655). Within this broad panorama of intervention, our review identified several developmental approaches as empirically and theoretically supported interventions for children with ASD.

In conclusion, this review showed different developmental therapies underlying the specific components in each of the approaches presented. Some of them are specifically implemented by the therapist, others are carried out by trained parents and/or teachers/educators. Some treatments focus on several developmental areas, others are focused on specific developmental areas, like joint attention. Some of them represent a combination of behavioral and developmental methods, others are more closely developmental approaches. This review also shows that a few of these methods require a comprehensive assessment as a prerequisite to calibrate the intervention. Additionally, despite its great significance, little attention is still given to early intervention for ASD, and the study of the effectiveness of these methods in long-term longitudinal studies. For future research it is also important to increase the number of individuals involved, focusing on different children's developmental ages, giving greater emphasis to the approaches with more significant effect sizes.

## REFERENCES


[1] American Psychiatric Association. 2013. *Diagnostic and statistical manual of mental disorders, 5th edition.* Author: Washington.

[2] Elsabbagh, M., Divan, G., Koh, Y. J., Kim, Y. S., Kauchali, S., Marcín, C., & Yasamy, M. T. 2012. "Global prevalence of autism and other pervasive developmental disorders." *Autism research* 5(3): 160-179. doi: 10.1002/aur.239.

[3] Tsai, L. Y. 2014. "Impact of DSM-5 on epidemiology of autism spectrum disorder." *Research in Autism Spectrum Disorders* 8(11): 1454-1470. doi: 10.1016/j.rasd.2014.07.016.

[4] American Psychiatric Association. 1994. *Diagnostic and statistical manual of mental disorders, 4th edition.* Washington, DC: Author.

[5] American Psychiatric Association. 2000. *Diagnostic and statistical manual of mental disorders, 4th edition, text revised.* Washington, DC: Author.

[6] Soldateschi M, Ambrosio V, Scattoni ML, Chiarotti F, Venerosi A. 2016.Tools for surveillance and care of children with autism spectrum disorder: the role of pediatricians in early recognition. ISTISAN reports 16/24. (Tr. It. *Strumenti per sorveglianza e presa in carico di bambini con disturbo dello spettro autistico: il ruolo dei pediatri nel riconoscimento precoce. Rapporti ISTISAN16/24.*). Retrived 05/10/2019 from http://old.iss.it/binary/publ/cont/16_24_web.pdf.

[7] Christensen, D. L., Maenner, M. J., Bilder, D., Constantino, J. N., Daniels, J., Durkin, M. S., & Shenouda, J. 2019. "Prevalence and Characteristics of Autism Spectrum Disorder Among Children Aged 4 Years—Early Autism and Developmental Disabilities Monitoring Network, Seven Sites, United States, 2010, 2012, and 2014." *MMWR Surveillance Summaries* 68(2): 1-58. doi: 10.15585/mmwr.ss6802a1.

[8] Baio, J., Wiggins, L., Christensen, D. L., Maenner, M. J., Daniels, J., Warren, Z., & Durkin, M. S. 2018. "Prevalence of autism spectrum disorder among children aged 8 years—autism and developmental disabilities monitoring network, 11 sites, United States, 2014." *MMWR Surveillance Summaries* 67(6): 1-23. doi: 10.15585/mmwr.ss6706a1.

[9] ASDEU 2018. "*Autism Spectrum Disorders in the European Union (ASDEU): final report: main results of the ASDEU project.*" Retrived 26/09/2019, from http://asdeu.eu/wp-content/uploads/2016/12/ASDEUExecSummary27September2018.pdf.

[10] Istat. 2018. "The integration of students with disabilities in primary and secondary schools" (Tr. it. *L'integrazione degli alunni con disabilità nelle scuole primarie e secondarie di primo grado*). Retrived 06/10/2019, from https://www.istat.it/it/files/2018/03/alunni-con-disabilit%C3%A0-as2016-2017.pdf.

[11] Narzisi, A., Posada, M., Barbieri, F., Chericoni, N., Ciuffolini, D., Pinzino, M., & Muratori, F. 2020. "Prevalence of autism spectrum disorder in a large Italian catchment area: a school-based population study within the ASDEU project." *Epidemiology and psychiatric sciences* 29. doi: 10.1017/S2045796018000483.

[12] Salomone, E., Beranová, Š., Bonnet-Brilhault, F., Briciet Lauritsen, M., Budisteanu, M., Buitelaar, J., & Fuentes, J. 2016. "Use of early intervention for young children with autism spectrum disorder across Europe." *Autism* 20(2): 233-249. doi: 10.1177/1362361315577218.

[13] Wagner A., Wallace K., Rogers S. 2014. "Developmental Approaches to Treatment of Young Children with Autism Spectrum Disorder." In Handbook of Early Intervention for Autism Spectrum Disorders. *Autism and Child Psychopathology Series*, edited by Tarbox J., Dixon D., Sturmey P., Matson J., 393-427. New York: Springer. doi: 10.1007/978-1-4939-0401-3_20.

[14] Beebe, B. 2017. "Daniel Stern: Microanalysis and the empirical infant research foundations." *Psychoanalytic Inquiry* 37(4): 228-241. doi: 10.1080/07351690.2017.1299498.

[15] Beebe, B., & Lachmann, F. M. 1988. "The contribution of mother-infant mutual influence to the origins of self- and object representations." *Psychoanalytic Psychology* 5(4): 305–337. doi: 10.1037/0736-9735.5.4.305.

[16] Cassidy, J., &, Shaver, P. R. (Eds.) 2016. *Handbook of Attachment, 3rd edition: Theory, Research, And Clinical Applications*. New York: Guilford Press.

[17] McKenzie, R., & Dallos, R. 2017. "Autism and attachment difficulties: Overlap of symptoms, implications and innovative solutions." *Clinical child psychology and psychiatry* 22(4): 632-648. doi: 10.1177/1359104517707323.

[18] Stern, D. N. 1998. *The motherhood constellation: A unified view of parent-infant psychotherapy.* London: Karnac books.

[19] Tronick, E., Als, H., Adamson, L., Wise, S., & Brazelton, T. B. 1978. "The infant's response to entrapment between contradictory messages in face-to-face interaction." *Journal of the American Academy of Child psychiatry* 17(1): 1-13. doi: 10.1016/S0002-7138(09)62273-1.

[20] LeBlanc, L. A., Riley, A. R., & Goldsmith, T. R. 2008. "Autism spectrum disorders: A lifespan perspective." In *Clinical assessment and intervention for autism spectrum disorders,* edited by J. L. Matson, 65-87. Burlington, MA: Academic Press.

[21] Greenspan, S. I., & Wieder, S. 1997. "Developmental patterns and outcomes in infants and children with disorders in relating and communicating: A chart review of 200 cases of children with autistic spectrum diagnoses." *Journal of Developmental and Learning Disorders* 1: 87-142.

[22] Siller, M., & Sigman, M. 2002. "The behaviors of parents of children with autism predict the subsequent development of their children's communication." *Journal of autism and developmental disorders* 32(2): 77-89. doi: 10.1023/A:1014884404276.

[23] Hillman, H. 2018. "Child-centered play therapy as an intervention for children with autism: A literature review." *International Journal of Play Therapy* 27(4): 198–204. doi: 10.1037/pla0000083.

[24] Lifter, K., Foster-Sanda, S., Arzamarski, C., Briesch, J., & McClure, E. 2011. "Overview of play: Its uses and importance in early intervention/early childhood special education." *Infants & Young Children* 24(3): 225-245. doi: 10.1097/IYC.0b013e31821e995c.

[25] Pittala, E. T., Saint-Georges-Chaumet, Y., Favrot, C., Tanet, A., Cohen, D., & Saint-Georges, C. 2018. "Clinical outcomes of interactive, intensive and individual (3i) play therapy for children with ASD: a two-year follow-up study." *BMC pediatrics* 18(1): 165-178. doi: 10.1186/s12887-018-1126-7.

[26] Di Renzo, M., di Castelbianco, F. B., Plescia, F., Racinaro, L., Petrillo, M., & Rea, M. 2016. "The understanding of others intentions can predict the improvement of symptomatology in children with autism– An exploratory study." *Current Pediatric Research* 20(2): 183-192.

[27] Schertz, H. H., Baker, C., Hurwitz, S., & Benner, L. 2011. "Principles of early intervention reflected in toddler research in autism spectrum disorders." *Topics in Early Childhood Special Education* 31(1): 4–21. doi: 10.1177/0271121410382460.

[28] Greenspan, S. I., & Wieder, S. 1999. "A functional developmental approach to autism spectrum disorders." *Journal of the Association for Persons with Severe Handicaps* 24(3): 147-161. doi: 10.2511/rpsd.24.3.147.

[29] Pajareya, K., & Nopmaneejumruslers, K. 2011. "A pilot randomized controlled trial of DIR/Floortime™ parent training intervention for pre-school children with autistic spectrum disorders." *Autism* 15(5): 563-577. doi: 10.1177/1362361310386502.

[30] Solomon, R., Necheles, J., Ferch, C., & Bruckman, D. 2007. "Pilot study of a parent training program for young children with autism: The PLAY Project Home Consultation program." *Autism* 11(3): 205-224. doi: 10.1177/1362361307076842.

[31] Mercer, J. 2017. "Examining DIR/Floortime™ as a treatment for children with autism spectrum disorders: A review of research and theory." *Research on Social Work Practice* 27(5): 625-635. doi: 10.1177/1049731515583062.

[32] Morgan, L. J., Rubin, E., Coleman, J. J., Frymark, T., Wang, B. P., & Cannon, L. J. 2014. "Impact of social communication interventions on infants and toddlers with or at-risk for autism: A systematic review." *Focus on Autism and Other Developmental Disabilities* 29(4): 246-256. doi: 10.1177/1088357614539835.

[33] Ayres A. J. 1979. *Sensory Integration and the Child.* Los Angeles, CA: Western Psychological Services.

[34] Green, M. D. A., Wachs, H., & Dee, M. 2014. "Successful optometric vision therapy with patients on the autistic spectrum: Engaging patients with visual-cognitive therapy." *Optometry & Visual Performance* 2(5): 235–239.

[35] Au, M., & Cuolter, R. 2014. "Vision therapy for the autistic patient: A literature review and case report." *Optometry & Visual Performance* 2: 244-250.

[36] Lawton, K., & Kasari, C. 2012. "Teacher-implemented joint attention intervention: Pilot randomized controlled study for preschoolers with autism." *Journal of consulting and clinical psychology* 80(4): 687-693. doi: 10.1037/a0028506.

[37] Kasari, C., Freeman, S., & Paparella, T. 2006. "Joint attention and symbolic play in young children with autism: A randomized controlled intervention study." *Journal of Child Psychology and Psychiatry* 47(6): 611-620. doi: 10.1111/j.1469-7610. 2005.01567.x.

[38] Goods, K. S., Ishijima, E., Chang, Y. C., & Kasari, C. 2013. "Preschool based JASPER intervention in minimally verbal children with autism: Pilot RCT." *Journal of autism and developmental disorders* 43(5): 1050-1056. doi: 10.1007/s10803-012-1644-3.

[39] Kasari, C., Gulsrud, A. C., Wong, C., Kwon, S., & Locke, J. 2010. "Randomized controlled caregiver mediated joint engagement intervention for toddlers with autism." *Journal of autism and developmental disorders* 40(9): 1045-1056. doi: 10.1007/s10803-010-0955-5.

[40] Kasari, C., Lawton, K., Shih, W., Barker, T. V., Landa, R., Lord, C., & Senturk, D. 2014a. "Caregiver-mediated intervention for low-

resourced preschoolers with autism: An RCT." *Pediatrics* 134(1): e72-e79. doi: 10.1542/peds.2013-3229.

[41] Kasari, C., Gulsrud, A., Paparella, T., Hellemann, G., & Berry, K. 2015. "Randomized comparative efficacy study of parent-mediated interventions for toddlers with autism." *Journal of consulting and clinical psychology* 83(3): 554. doi: 10.1037/a0039080.

[42] Chang, Y. C., Shire, S. Y., Shih, W., Gelfand, C., & Kasari, C. 2016. "Preschool deployment of evidence-based social communication intervention: JASPER in the classroom." *Journal of autism and developmental disorders* 46(6): 2211-2223. doi: 10.1007/s10803-016-2752-2.

[43] Shire, S. Y., Chang, Y. C., Shih, W., Bracaglia, S., Kodjoe, M., & Kasari, C. 2017. "Hybrid implementation model of community-partnered early intervention for toddlers with autism: A randomized trial." *Journal of Child Psychology and Psychiatry* 58(5): 612–622. doi: 10.1111/jcpp.12672.

[44] Shire, S. Y., Shih, W., Chang, Y. C., Bracaglia, S., Kodjoe, M., & Kasari, C. 2019. "Sustained Community Implementation of JASPER Intervention with Toddlers with Autism." *Journal of autism and developmental disorders* 49(5): 1863-1875. doi: 10.1007/s10803-018-03875-0.

[45] Chang, Y. C., Shih, W., Landa, R., Kaiser, A., & Kasari, C. 2018. "Symbolic play in school-aged minimally verbal children with autism spectrum disorder." *Journal of autism and developmental disorders* 48(5): 1436-1445. doi: 10.1007/s10803-017-3388-6.

[46] Almirall, D., DiStefano, C., Chang, Y. C., Shire, S., Kaiser, A., Lu, X., & Kasari, C. 2016. "Longitudinal effects of adaptive interventions with a speech-generating device in minimally verbal children with ASD." *Journal of Clinical Child & Adolescent Psychology* 45(4): 442-456. doi: 10.1080/15374416.2016.1138407.

[47] Dawson, G., Rogers, S., Munson, J., Smith, M., Winter, J., Greenson, J., & Varley, J. 2010. "Randomized, controlled trial of an intervention for toddlers with autism: the Early Start Denver Model." *Pediatrics* 125(1): e17-e23. doi: 10.1542/peds.2009-0958.

[48] Vivanti, G., Dissanayake, C., Zierhut, C., Rogers, S. J., & Victorian ASELCC Team. 2013. "Brief report: Predictors of outcomes in the Early Start Denver Model delivered in a group setting." *Journal of Autism and Developmental Disorders* 43(7): 1717-1724. doi: 10.1007/s10803-012-1705-7.

[49] Zhou, B., Xu, Q., Li, H., Zhang, Y., Wang, Y., Rogers, S. J., & Xu, X. 2018. "Effects of parent-implemented Early Start Denver Model intervention on Chinese Toddlers with autism spectrum disorder: A non-randomized controlled trial." *Autism Research* 11(4): 654-666. doi: 10.1002/aur.1917.

[50] Dawson, G., Jones, E. J., Merkle, K., Venema, K., Lowy, R., Faja, S., & Smith, M. 2012. "Early behavioral intervention is associated with normalized brain activity in young children with autism." *Journal of the American Academy of Child & Adolescent Psychiatry* 51(11): 1150-1159. doi: 10.1016/j.jaac.2012.08.018.

[51] Estes, A., Munson, J., Rogers, S. J., Greenson, J., Winter, J., & Dawson, G. 2015. "Long-term outcomes of early intervention in 6-year-old children with autism spectrum disorder." *Journal of the American Academy of Child & Adolescent Psychiatry* 54(7): 580-587. doi: 10.1016/j.jaac.2015.04.005.

[52] Rogers, S. J., Estes, A., Lord, C., Munson, J., Rocha, M., Winter, J., & Sugar, C. A. 2019. "A multisite randomized controlled two-phase trial of the early Start Denver Model compared to treatment as usual." *Journal of the American Academy of Child & Adolescent Psychiatry* 58(9): 853-865. doi: 10.1016/j.jaac.2019.01.004.

[53] Waddington, H., van der Meer, L., & Sigafoos, J. 2016. "Erratum to: Effectiveness of the Early Start Denver Model: a Systematic Review." *Review Journal of Autism and Developmental Disorders* 3(4): 399-399. doi: 10.1007/s40489-016-0095-8.

[54] Rogers, S. J., Estes, A., Vismara, L., Munson, J., Zierhut, C., Greenson, J., & Whelan, F. 2019. "Enhancing low-intensity coaching in parent implemented Early Start Denver Model intervention for early autism: A randomized comparison treatment trial." *Journal of*

*autism and developmental disorders* 49(2): 632-646. doi: 10.1007/s10803-018-3740-5.

[55] 55.Capes, K., Upson, S., Jones, C., Dissanayake, C., & Vivanti, G. 2019. "Delivery of Group-Early Start Denver Model in an Australian early childhood setting." *Pediatric Medicine* 2: 16-25. doi: 10.21037/pm.2019.04.04.

[56] Vivanti, G., Dissanayake, C., Duncan, E., Feary, J., Capes, K., Upson, S., & Hudry, K. 2019. "Outcomes of children receiving Group-Early Start Denver Model in an inclusive versus autism-specific setting: A pilot randomized controlled trial." *Autism* 23(5): 1165-1175. doi: 10.1177/1362361318801341.

[57] Hart, B., & Risley, T. R. 1975. "Incidental teaching of language in the preschool." *Journal of applied behavior analysis* 8(4): 411-420. doi: 10.1901/jaba.1975.8-411.

[58] Franco, J. H., Davis, B. L., & Davis, J. L. 2013. "Increasing social interaction using prelinguistic milieu teaching with nonverbal school-age children with autism." *American Journal of Speech-Language Pathology* 22(3): 489-502. doi: 10.1044/1058-0360(2012/10-0103).

[59] Hancock, T. B., & Kaiser, A. P. 2006. "Enhanced Milieu Teaching." In *Treatment of Language Disorders in Children*, edited by R. McCauley & M. Fey, 203-233. Baltimore: Paul Brookes.

[60] Fey, M. E., Warren, S. F., Brady, N., Finestack, L. H., Bredin-Oja, S. L., Fairchild, M., & Yoder, P. J. 2006. "Early effects of responsivity education/prelinguistic milieu teaching for children with developmental delays and their parents." *Journal of Speech, Language, and Hearing Research* 49(3): 526-547. doi: 10.1044/ 1092-4388(2006/039).

[61] Yoder, P. J., & Warren, S. F. 1998. "Maternal responsivity predicts the prelinguistic communication intervention that facilitates generalized intentional communication." *Journal of Speech, Language, and Hearing Research* 41: 1207–1219. doi: 10.1044/jslhr.4105.1207.

[62] Christensen-Sandfort, R. J., & Whinnery, S. B. 2013. "Impact of milieu teaching on communication skills of young children with

autism spectrum disorder." *Topics in Early Childhood Special Education* 32(4): 211-222. doi: 10.1177/0271121411404930.

[63] Dubin, A. H., Lieberman-Betz, R. G., Ayres, K. M., & Zawoyski, A. 2019. "The Effects of Prelinguistic Milieu Teaching Implemented in Classrooms for Preschoolers With or at Risk for Autism Spectrum Disorder." *Focus on Autism and Other Developmental Disabilities*. doi: 10.1177/1088357619888917.

[64] Peters-Scheffer, N. C., Huskens, B., Didden, R., & van der Meer, L. 2016. "Prelinguistic milieu teaching." In *Early intervention for young children with autism spectrum disorder,* edited by R. Lang, T. B. Hancock and N. N. Singh, 151-175. Cham, Switzerland: Springer International Publishing.

[65] Yoder, P. J., & Lieberman, R. G. 2010. "Brief report: randomized test of the efficacy of picture exchange communication system on highly generalized picture exchanges in children with ASD." *Journal of autism and developmental disorders* 40(5): 629-632. doi: 10.1007/s10803-009-0897-y.

[66] Mcduffie, A. S., Lieberman, R. G., & Yoder, P. J. 2012. "Object interest in autism spectrum disorder: A treatment comparison." *Autism* 16(4): 398-405. doi: 10.1177/1362361309360983.

[67] Kaiser, A. P., & Roberts, M. Y. 2013. "Parent-implemented enhanced milieu teaching with preschool children who have intellectual disabilities." *Journal of Speech, Language, and Hearing Research* 56(1): 295-309. doi: 10.1044/1092-4388(2012/11-0231).

[68] Kasari, C., Kaiser, A., Goods, K., Nietfeld, J., Mathy, P., Landa, R., & Almirall, D. 2014. "Communication interventions for minimally verbal children with autism: A sequential multiple assignment randomized trial." *Journal of the American Academy of Child & Adolescent Psychiatry* 53(6): 635-646. doi: 10.1016/j.jaac. 2014.01.019.

[69] Hampton, L. H., Harty, M., Fuller, E. A., & Kaiser, A. P. 2019. "Enhanced milieu teaching for children with autism spectrum disorder in South Africa." *International journal of speech-language pathology* 21(6): 1-11. doi: 10.1080/17549507.2018.1559357.

[70] Mancil, G. R. 2009. "Milieu therapy as a communication intervention: A review of the literature related to children with autism spectrum disorder." *Education and Training in Developmental Disabilities* 44(1): 105-117.

[71] Parker-McGowan, Q., Chen, M., Reichle, J., Pandit, S., Johnson, L., & Kreibich, S. 2014. "Describing treatment intensity in milieu teaching interventions for children with developmental disabilities: A review." *Language, speech, and hearing services in schools* 45(4): 351-364. doi: 10.1044/2014_LSHSS-13-0087.

[72] Mesibov, G. B., Shea, V., & Schopler, E. 2005. *The TEACCH approach to autism spectrum disorders.* New York: Springer Science & Business Media.

[73] Mesibov, G. B., & Shea, V. 2010. "The TEACCH program in the era of evidence-based practice." *Journal of autism and developmental disorders* 40(5): 570-579. doi: 10.1007/s10803-009-0901-6.

[74] Van Bourgondien M. E., Coonrod E. 2013. "TEACCH: An Intervention Approach for Children and Adults with Autism Spectrum Disorders and their Families." In *Interventions for Autism Spectrum Disorders*, edited by Goldstein S., Naglieri J., 75-105. New York: Springer. doi: 10.1007/978-1-4614-5301-7_5.

[75] Virués-Ortega J., Arnold-Saritepe A., Hird C., Phillips K. 2017. "The TEACCH Program for People with Autism: Elements, Outcomes, and Comparison with Competing Models." In *Handbook of Treatments for Autism Spectrum Disorder. Autism and Child Psychopathology Series*, edited by Matson J., 427–436. Cham, Switzerland: Springer International Publishing. doi: 10.1007/978-3-319-61738-1_23.

[76] Schopler, E., & Reichler, R. J. 1971. "Parents as cotherapists in the treatment of psychotic children." *Journal of autism and childhood schizophrenia* 1(1): 87-102. doi: 10.1007/BF01537746.

[77] Virues-Ortega, J., Julio, F. M., & Pastor-Barriuso, R. 2013. "The TEACCH program for children and adults with autism: A meta-analysis of intervention studies." *Clinical psychology review* 33(8): 940-953. doi: 10.1016/j.cpr.2013.07.005.

[78] Callahan, K., Shukla-Mehta, S., Magee, S., & Wie, M. 2010. "ABA versus TEACCH: the case for defining and validating comprehensive treatment models in autism." *Journal of autism and developmental disorders* 40(1): 74-88. doi: 10.1007/s10803-009-0834-0.

[79] Ichikawa, K., Takahashi, Y., Ando, M., Anme, T., Ishizaki, T., Yamaguchi, H., & Nakayama, T. 2013. "TEACCH-based group social skills training for children with high-functioning autism: a pilot randomized controlled trial." *BioPsychoSocial medicine* 7(1): 14-22. doi:10.1186/1751-0759-7-14.

[80] Coman, D., Alessandri, M., Gutierrez, A., Novotny, S., Boyd, B., Hume, K., & Odom, S. 2013. "Commitment to classroom model philosophy and burnout symptoms among high fidelity teachers implementing preschool programs for children with autism spectrum disorders." *Journal of autism and developmental disorders* 43(2): 345-360. doi: 10.1007/s10803-012-1573-1.

[81] Boyd, B. A., Hume, K., McBee, M. T., Alessandri, M., Gutierrez, A., Johnson, L., & Odom, S. L. 2014. "Comparative efficacy of LEAP, TEACCH and non-model-specific special education programs for preschoolers with autism spectrum disorders." *Journal of autism and developmental disorders* 44(2): 366-380. doi: 10.1007/s10803-013-1877-9.

[82] Aoyama, S. 1995. "The efficacy of structuring the work system: Individualization of the work format and the use of a 3-level paper rack in a special education class." *Japanese Journal of Special Education* 32(5): 1–5.

[83] Ozonoff, S., & Cathcart, K. 1998. "Effectiveness of a home program intervention for young children with autism." *Journal of Autism and Developmental Disorders* 28: 25–32. doi: https://doi.org/10.1023/A:1026006818310.

[84] Persson, B. 2000. "Brief report: A longitudinal study of quality of life and independence among adult men with autism." *Journal of Autism and Developmental Disorders* 30: 61–66. doi: 10.1023/a:1005464128544.

[85] Panerai, S., Ferrante, L., & Zingale, M. 2002. "Benefits of the Treatment and Education of Autistic and Communication Handicapped Children (TEACCH) programme as compared with a non-specific approach." *Journal of Intellectual Disability Research* 46: 318–327. doi: 10.1046/j.1365-2788.2002.00388.x.

[86] Van Bourgondien,M. E., Reichle, N. C., & Schopler, E. 2003. "Effects of amodel treatment approach on adults with autism." *Journal of Autism and Developmental Disorders* 33: 131–140. doi: 10.1023/A:1022931224934.

[87] Siaperas, P., & Beadle-Brown, J. 2006. "A case study of the use of a structured teaching approach in adults with autism in a residential home in Greece." *Autism* 10: 330–343. doi: 10.1177/1362361 306064433.

[88] Siaperas, P., Higgins, S., & Proios, P. 2007. "Challenging behaviours on people with autism: A case study on the effect of a residential training programme based on structured teaching and TEACCH method." *Psychiatriki* 18(4): 343–350.

[89] Tsang, S., Shek, D., Lam, L., Tang, F., & Cheung, P. 2007. "Brief report: Application of the TEACCH program on Chinese pre-school children with autism — Does culture make a difference?" *Journal of Autism and Developmental Disorders* 37: 390–396. doi: 10.1007/ s10803-006-0199-6.

[90] Probst, P., & Leppert, T. 2008. "Brief report: Outcomes of a teacher training program for autism spectrum disorders." *Journal of Autism and Developmental Disorders* 38: 1791–1796. doi: 10.1007/s10803-008-0561-y.

[91] Panerai, S., Zingale, M., Trubia, G., Finocchiaro, M., Zuccarello, R., Ferrei, R., et al. 2009. "Special education versus inclusive education: The TEACCH program." *Journal of Autism and Developmental Disorders* 39: 874–882. doi: 10.1007/s10803-009-0696-5.

[92] McConkey, R., Truesdale-Kennedy, M., Crawford, H., McGreevy, E., Reavey,M., & Cassidy, A. 2010. "Preschoolers with autism spectrum disorders: Evaluating the impact of a home-based intervention to

promote their communication." *Early Child Development & Care* 180: 299–315. doi: 10.1080/03004430801899187.

[93] Braiden, H. J., McDaniel, B., McCrudden, E., Hanes, M., & Crozier, B. 2012. "A practice-based evaluation of Barnardo's forward steps early intervention programme for children diagnosed with autism." *Child Care in Practice* 18: 227–242. doi: 10.1080/13575279. 2012.683773.

[94] Welterlin, A., Turner-Brown, L. M., Harris, S., Mesibov, G., & Delmolino, L. 2012. "The home TEACCHing program for toddlers with autism." *Journal of Autism and Developmental Disorders* 42: 1827–1835. doi: 10.1007/s10803-011-1419-2.

[95] Turner-Brown, L., Hume, K., Boyd, B. A., & Kainz, K. 2019. "Preliminary efficacy of family implemented TEACCH for toddlers: effects on parents and their toddlers with autism spectrum disorder." *Journal of Autism and Developmental Disorders* 49(7): 2685-2698. doi: 10.1007/s10803-016-2812-7.

[96] Carter, A. S., Messinger, D. S., Stone, W. L., Celimli, S., Nahmias, A. S., & Yoder, P. 2011. "A randomized controlled trial of Hanen's 'More Than Words' in toddlers with early autism symptoms." *Journal of Child Psychology and Psychiatry* 52(7): 741-752. doi: 10.1111/j.1469-7610.2011.02395.x.

[97] Weitzman, E. 2013. "More than words—The Hanen Program for parents of children with autism spectrum disorder: A teaching model for parent-implemented language intervention." *Perspectives on Language Learning and Education* 20(3): 96-111. doi: 10.1044/lle20.3.86.

[98] Prelock, P. A., Calhoun, J., Morris, H., & Platt, G. 2011. "Supporting parents to facilitate communication and joint attention in their young children with autism spectrum disorders: Two pilot studies." *Topics in Language Disorders* 31(3): 210-234. doi: 10.1097/TLD. 0b013e318227bd3f.

[99] Zaman, T., Das, D., & Chowdhury, M. A. 2017. "Outcomes of An Early Intervention Programme on Children with Autism Spectrum

Disorders." *Chattagram Maa-O-Shishu Hospital Medical College Journal* 16(2): 9-13. doi: 10.3329/cmoshmcj.v16i2.37285.

[100] Sokmun, S., Singh, S. J., & Vandort, S. 2018. "The impact of Hanen More Than Words programme on parents of children with ASD in Malaysia." *Jurnal Sains Kesihatan Malaysia (Malaysian Journal of Health Sciences)* 15(2): 43-51. doi: 10.17576/JSKM-2017-1502-06.

[101] Green, J., Charman, T., McConachie, H., Aldred, C., Slonims, V., Howlin, P., & Barrett, B. (2010). "Parent-mediated communication-focused treatment in children with autism (PACT): a randomised controlled trial." *The Lancet* 375(9732): 2152-2160. doi: 10.1016/S0140-6736(10)60587-9.

[102] Green, J., & Garg, S. 2018. "Annual Research Review: the state of autism intervention science: progress, target psychological and biological mechanisms and future prospects." *Journal of Child Psychology and Psychiatry* 59(4): 424-443. doi: 10.1111/jcpp.12892.

[103] Pickles, A., Harris, V., Green, J., Aldred, C., McConachie, H., Slonims, V., & PACT Consortium. 2015. "Treatment mechanism in the MRC preschool autism communication trial: Implications for study design and parent-focussed therapy for children." *Journal of Child Psychology and Psychiatry* 56(2): 162-170. doi: 10.1111/jcpp.12291.

[104] Pickles, A., Le Couteur, A., Leadbitter, K., Salomone, E., Cole-Fletcher, R., Tobin, H., & Aldred, C. 2016. "Parent-mediated social communication therapy for young children with autism (PACT): long-term follow-up of a randomised controlled trial." *The Lancet* 388(10059): 2501-2509. doi: 10.1016/S0140-6736(16)31229-6.

[105] Rahman, A., Divan, G., Hamdani, S. U., Vajaratkar, V., Taylor, C., Leadbitter, K., & Patel, V. 2016. "Effectiveness of the parent-mediated intervention for children with autism spectrum disorder in south Asia in India and Pakistan (PASS): a randomised controlled trial." *The Lancet Psychiatry* 3(2): 128-136. doi: 10.1016/S2215-0366(15)00388-0.

[106] Salomone, E., Leadbitter, K., Aldred, C., Barrett, B., Byford, S., Charman, T., & Parr, J. R. 2018. "The association between child and

family characteristics and the mental health and wellbeing of caregivers of children with autism in mid-childhood." *Journal of autism and developmental disorders* 48(4): 1189-1198. doi: 10.1007/s10803-017-3392-x.

[107] Schertz, H. H., Odom, S. L., Baggett, K. M., & Sideris, J. H. 2013. "Effects of joint attention mediated learning for toddlers with autism spectrum disorders: An initial randomized controlled study." *Early Childhood Research Quarterly* 28(2): 249-258. doi: 10.1016/j. ecresq.2012.06.006.

[108] Klein, P. S. 2003. "A mediational approach to early intervention: Israel." In *Early intervention practices around the world*, edited by S .L. Odom, M. J. Hanson, J. A. Blackman & S. Kaul, 69–80. Baltimore: Paul H. Brookes.

[109] Lee, K., & Schertz, H. H. 2019. "Brief Report: Analysis of the Relationship Between Turn Taking and Joint Attention for Toddlers with Autism." *Journal of autism and developmental disorders*, 1-8. doi: 10.1007/s10803-019-03979-1.

[110] Schertz, H. H., Odom, S. L., Baggett, K. M., & Sideris, J. H. 2018. "Mediating parent learning to promote social communication for toddlers with autism: Effects from a randomized controlled trial." *Journal of autism and developmental disorders* 48(3): 853-867. doi: 10.1007/s10803-017-3386-8.

[111] Di Renzo, M., ed. 2020. "The developmental-relational approch to autism" (Tr. It. *L'approccio evolutivo-relazionale all'autismo*). Roma: Edizioni Magi.

[112] Greenspan, S. I. 2001. "The affect diathesis hypothesis: The role of emotions in the core deficit in autism and in the development of intelligence and social skills." *Journal of Developmental and Learning Disorders* 5(1): 1-45.

[113] Di Renzo, M., Bianchi di Castelbianco, F., Vanadia, E., Petrillo, M., Racinaro, L., & Rea, M. 2016. "From the emotional integration to the cognitive construction: The developmental approach of turtle project in children with autism spectrum disorder." *Autism-Open Access* 6: 160-169. doi: 10.4172/2165-7890.1000160.

[114] Di Renzo, M., Bianchi di Castelbianco, F., Vanadia, E., Petrillo, M., Racinaro, L., & Rea, M. 2016. "TULIP Protocol (TCE, UOI, Leiter-R as Indicators of Predictivity) for the Assessment of the Developmental Potential in Children with Autism Spectrum Disorders." *Autism Open Access* 6(4): 188-194. doi: 10.4172/2165-7890.1000188.

[115] Istituto Di Ortofonologia. 2016. "Holophony. Three-dimensional listening for a new therapeutic model" (Tr. It. *Olofonia. L'ascolto tridimensionale per un nuovo modello terapeutico*). Roma: Edizioni Magi.

[116] Di Renzo, M., di Castelbianco, F. B., Vanadia, E., Petrillo, M., Racinaro, L., Stracqualursi, M., & Rea, M. 2016. "Assessment of executive functions in preschool-aged children with autism spectrum disorders: Usefulness and limitation of BRIEF-P in clinical practice." *Journal of Child and Adolescent Behavior* 4(5): 313-20. doi: 10.4172/2375-4494.1000313.

[117] Di Renzo, M., Guerriero, V., Petrillo, M., Racinaro, L., Vanadia, E., & Bianchi di Castelbianco, F. 2019. "A comprehensive assessment process for children with autism spectrum disorders." *Advances in Autism* 1-13. doi: 10.1108/AIA-09-2018-0031.

[118] Di Renzo, M., Di Castelbianco, F. B., Petrillo, M., Racinaro, L., & Rea, M. 2015. "Assessment of a long-term developmental relationship-based approach in children with autism spectrum disorder." *Psychological reports* 117(1): 26-49. doi: 10.2466/15.10.PR0.117c15z8.

[119] Di Renzo, M. 2017. "The Theoretical Principles of the Body-Centered Therapy to Promote Affective Attunement in Children with Autism Spectrum Disorder." *Journal of Behavioral and Brain Science* 7(12): 545-556. doi: 10.4236/jbbs.2017.712039.

[120] Ingersoll, B., & Dvortcsak, A. 2010. *Teaching social communication to children with autism: A practicioner's guide to parent training.* New York, NY: The Guilford.

[121] Ingersoll, B., & Wainer, A. 2013. "Initial efficacy of Project ImPACT: A parent-mediated social communication intervention for young

children with ASD." *Journal of autism and developmental disorders* 43(12): 2943-2952. doi: 10.1007/s10803-013-1840-9.

[122] Stadnick, N. A., Stahmer, A., & Brookman-Frazee, L. 2015. "Preliminary effectiveness of project ImPACT: A parent-mediated intervention for children with autism spectrum disorder delivered in a community program." *Journal of autism and developmental disorders* 45(7): 2092-2104. doi: 10.1007/s10803-015-2376-y.

[123] Rieth, S. R., Haine-Schlagel, R., Burgeson, M., Searcy, K., Dickson, K. S., & Stahmer, A. C. 2018. "Integrating a Parent-Implemented Blend of Developmental and Behavioral Intervention Strategies into Speech-Language Treatment for Toddlers at Risk for Autism Spectrum Disorder." *Seminars in speech and language* 39(2): 114-124. doi: 10.1055/s-0038-1627483.

[124] Stahmer, A. C., Rieth, S. R., Dickson, K. S., Feder, J., Burgeson, M., Searcy, K., & Brookman-Frazee, L. 2019. "Project ImPACT for Toddlers: Pilot outcomes of a community adaptation of an intervention for autism risk." *Autism.* doi: 10.1177/136236131 9878080.

[125] Manohar, H., Kandasamy, P., Chandrasekaran, V., & Rajkumar, R. P. 2019. "Brief Parent-Mediated Intervention for Children with Autism Spectrum Disorder: A Feasibility Study from South India." *Journal of autism and developmental disorders* 49: 1-13. doi: 10.1007/s10803-019-04032-x.

[126] Kasari, C., Gulsrud, A., Freeman, S., Paparella, T., & Hellemann, G. 2012. "Longitudinal follow-up of children with autism receiving targeted interventions on joint attention and play." *Journal of the American Academy of Child & Adolescent Psychiatry* 51(5): 487-495. doi: 10.1016/j.jaac.2012.02.019.

[127] Rollins, P. R., Campbell, M., Hoffman, R. T., & Self, K. 2016. "A community-based early intervention program for toddlers with autism spectrum disorders." Autism 20(2): 219-232. doi: 10.1177/ 1362361315577217.

[128] Rollins, P. R. 2017. "Pathways early intervention program for toddlers with autism." *Journal of Mental Health and Clinical Psychology* 1(1): 14-18. doi: 10.29245/2578/-2959/2018.1.1104.

[129] Rollins, P. R., John, S., Jones, A., & De Froy, A. 2019. "Pathways Early ASD Intervention as a Moderator of Parenting Stress on Parenting Behaviors: A Randomized Control Trial." *Journal of autism and developmental disorders* 49(10): 4280-4293. doi: 10.1007/s10803-019-04144-4.

[130] Gutstein, S. 2001. *Solving the relationship puzzle*. Arlington, TX: Future Horizons.

[131] Gutstein, S. E., Burgess, A. F., & Montfort, K. 2007. "Evaluation of the relationship development intervention program." *Autism* 11(5): 397-411. doi: 10.1177/1362361307079603.

[132] Wang, N., Wang, Y., & Han, H. 2019. "Efficiency of Relational Development Intervention Program for Children with Autism." *Advances in Social Science, Education and Humanities Research (ASSEHR)* 300. doi: 10.2991/erss-18.2019.163.

[133] Mahoney, G., & MacDonald, J. 2007. *Autism and developmental delays in young children: The responsive teaching curriculum for parents and professionals*. Austin, TX: Pro-Ed.

[134] Karaaslan, O., Diken, I. H., & Mahoney, G. 2013. "A randomized control study of responsive teaching with young Turkish children and their mothers." *Topics in Early Childhood Special Education* 33(1): 18-27. doi: 10.1177/0271121411429749.

[135] Mahoney, G., Wiggers, B., Nam, S., Kralovic, S., & Perales, F. 2014. "How depressive symptomatology of mothers of children with pervasive developmental disorders relates to their participation in relationship focused intervention." *International Journal of Early Childhood Special Education* 6(2): 204-221. doi: 10.20489/intjecse.86233.

[136] Alquraini, T., Al-Odaib, A., Al-Dhalaan, H., Merza, H., & Mahoney, G. 2019. "Relationship-based Intervention with Young Children with Autism in Saudi Arabia: Impediments and Consequences of Parenting Stress and Depression." *International Journal of Disability,*

*Development and Education* 66(3): 233-248. doi: 10.1080/1034912X.2018.1487042.

[137] Poslawsky, I. E., Naber, F. B., Bakermans-Kranenburg, M. J., De Jonge, M. V., Van Engeland, H., & Van IJzendoorn, M. H. 2014. "Development of a Video-feedback Intervention to promote Positive Parenting for Children with Autism (VIPP-AUTI)." *Attachment & Human Development* 16(4): 343-355. doi: 10.1080/14616734.2014.912487.

[138] Juffer, F. Bakermans-Kranenburg, M. J. & Van IJzendoorn, M. H. (Ed.). 2008. *Promoting positive parenting: An attachment-based intervention*. New York, NY: Lawrence Erlbaum Associates.

[139] Poslawsky, I. E., Naber, F. B., Bakermans-Kranenburg, M. J., van Daalen, E., van Engeland, H., & van IJzendoorn, M. H. 2015. "Video-feedback Intervention to promote Positive Parenting adapted to Autism (VIPP-AUTI): A randomized controlled trial." *Autism* 19(5): 588-603. doi: 10.1177/1362361314537124.

[140] Solomon, R., Van Egeren, L. A., Mahoney, G., Huber, M. S. Q., & Zimmerman, P. 2014. "PLAY Project Home Consultation intervention program for young children with autism spectrum disorders: a randomized controlled trial." *Journal of Developmental and Behavioral Pediatrics* 35(8): 475–485. doi: 10.1097/DBP.0000000000000096.

[141] Mahoney, G., & Solomon, R. 2016. "Mechanism of developmental change in the PLAY project home consultation program: Evidence from a randomized control trial." *Journal of autism and developmental disorders* 46(5): 1860-1871. doi: 10.1007/s10803-016-2720-x.

## BIOGRAPHICAL SKETCHES

### *Magda di Renzo*

**Affiliation:** Institute of Ortofonologia (IdO) in Rome, Italy

**Education:** MD in Philosophy, Speech Therapy and Psychology. Jungian analyst.

**Research and Professional Experience:** Since 1974 she has been carrying out clinical activities and teaching in the field of developmental pathologies. Her research interests concern developmental psychopathology, and especially on autism.

**Professional appointments**: Head of the Child and Adolescent Psychotherapy clinical service of the Institute of Ortofonologia (IdO). Member of CIPA (Italian Center for Analytical Psychology) and IAAP (International Association for Analytical Psychology).

**Publications from the Last 3 Years:**

1. Di Renzo, M., Guerriero, V., Petrillo, M., Racinaro, L., Vanadia, E., & di Castelbianco, F. B. (2019). A comprehensive assessment process for children with autism spectrum disorders. *Advances in Autism.*
2. Di Renzo, M. (2017). The Theoretical Principles of the Body-Centered Therapy to Promote Affective Attunement in Children with Autism Spectrum Disorder. *Journal of Behavioral and Brain Science*, *7*(12), 545.
3. Di Renzo, M., Bianchi di Castelbianco, F. B., Vanadia, E., & Racinaro, L. (2017). The psychomotor profile in children with autistic spectrum disorders: clinical assessments and implications for therapy. *Autism Open Access*, *7*(209), 2.
4. Di Renzo, M., Marini, C., Bianchi di Castelbianco, F., Racinaro, L., & Rea, M. (2017). Correlations between the Drawing Process in Autistic Children and Developmental Indexes. *J Psychol Psychother*, *7*(291), 2161-0487.
5. Di Renzo, M., Bianchi di Castelbianco, F., Vanadia, E., Petrillo, M., Racinaro, L., & Rea, M. (2017). Sensory processing and repetitive behaviors in clinical assessment of preschool children with autism

spectrum disorder. *Journal of Child and Adolescent Behavior*, *5*(2), 1-8.

6. Renzo, M. D., Palladino, G., & Bianchi di Castelbianco F., Racinaro L. (2017). When the Intellectual Potential is Concealed from Symptoms: A Case Report. *Journal of Clinical Case Report*, *7*(943), 2.

### *Viviana Guerriero*

**Affiliation:** Institute of Ortofonologia (IdO) in Rome, Italy

**Education:** PhD, Clinical psychology, and Psychotherapist.

**Research and Professional Experience:** In the research field she mainly works within the framework of attachment theory. In this area she participated in studies about parenting and couple relationships. She is currently investigating psychological experiences of adopted children/adolescents and their mothers, and children diagnosed with serious diseases and their parents. Her private practice as psychotherapist is focused on children, parents and young adults.

**Publications from the Last 3 Years:**

1. Pace, C. S., Guerriero, V., & Zavattini, G. C. (2020). Children's attachment representations: A pilot study comparing family drawing with narrative and behavioral assessments in adopted and community children. *The Arts in Psychotherapy*, *67*, 101612.
2. Pace, C. S., Di Folco, S., Guerriero, V., & Muzi, S. (2019). Late-adopted children grown up: a long-term longitudinal study on attachment patterns of adolescent adoptees and their adoptive mothers. *Attachment & human development*, *21*(4), 372-388.
3. Di Renzo, M., Guerriero, V., Petrillo, M., Racinaro, L., Vanadia, E., & di Castelbianco, F. B. (2019). A comprehensive assessment process for children with autism spectrum disorders. *Advances in Autism.*

4. de Campora, G., Giromini, L., Guerriero, V., Chiodo, C., Zavattini, G. C., & Larciprete, G. (2019). Influence of maternal reflective functioning on mothers' and children's weight: A follow-up study. *Infant Mental Health Journal*, *40*(6), 862-873.
5. Pace, C. S., Di Folco, S., & Guerriero, V. (2018). Late-adoptions in adolescence: Can attachment and emotion regulation influence behaviour problems? A controlled study using a moderation approach. *Clinical psychology & psychotherapy*, *25*(2), 250-262.
6. Guerriero V., de Campora G., Gnazzo A., Vegni E., Zavattini G. C. (2017). Parents facing their child disease: insights from attachment theory. In Alexandra M. Columbus (Eds.), *Advances in Psychology Research* (Vol. 126). Nova Science Publishers.

## *Valeria Mammarella*

**Affiliation:** Sapienza University of Rome

**Education:** MD in Medicine and Surgery

**Research and Professional Experience:** General practitioner substitute, Medical doctor, Specializing in Child neurology and psychiatry.

## *Federico Bianchi di Castelbianco*

**Affiliation:** Institute of Ortofonologia (IdO) in Rome, Italy

**Education:** MD in Psychology, Developmental psychotherapist.

**Research and Professional Experience:** His research interests focus on developmental psychopathology, and especially on Autism Spectrum Disorders.

**Professional Appointments:** Head of the Institute of Ortofonologia (IdO), Honorary Member of the Italian Society of Pediatry (SIP).

**Publications from the Last 3 Years:**

1. Di Renzo, M., Guerriero, V., Petrillo, M., Racinaro, L., Vanadia, E., & di Castelbianco, F. B. (2019). A comprehensive assessment process for children with autism spectrum disorders. *Advances in Autism.*
2. Di Renzo, M., Bianchi di Castelbianco, F. B., Vanadia, E., & Racinaro, L. (2017). The psychomotor profile in children with autistic spectrum disorders: clinical assessments and implications for therapy. *Autism Open Access*, *7*(209), 2.
3. Di Renzo, M., Marini, C., Bianchi di Castelbianco, F., Racinaro, L., & Rea, M. (2017). Correlations between the Drawing Process in Autistic Children and Developmental Indexes. *J Psychol Psychother*, *7*(291), 2161-0487.
4. Di Renzo, M., Bianchi di Castelbianco, F., Vanadia, E., Petrillo, M., Racinaro, L., & Rea, M. (2017). Sensory processing and repetitive behaviors in clinical assessment of preschool children with autism spectrum disorder. *Journal of Child and Adolescent Behavior*, *5*(2), 1-8.
5. Renzo, M. D., Palladino, G., & Bianchi di Castelbianco F., Racinaro L. (2017). When the Intellectual Potential is Concealed from Symptoms: A Case Report. *Journal of Clinical Case Report*, *7*(943), 2.

In: Understanding Children with Autism … ISBN: 978-1-53617-647-6
Editor: Anne Bourque 

*Chapter 4*

# EXPLORING THE PEDIATRIC VOLITION AMONG BOYS WITH AUTISM IN AN ADAPTED ROBOTICS PROGRAM

***Suk Young Hong*[1,*]*, Shannon Scratch*[1,2,3]*,***
***Fiona Moola*[1,2,5] *and Sally Lindsay*[1,2,4]**
[1]Rehabilitation Sciences Institute, University of Toronto,
Toronto, Ontario, Canada
[2]Bloorview Research Institute,
Holland Bloorview Kids Rehabilitation Hospital,
Toronto, Ontario, Canada
[3]Department of Pediatrics, University of Toronto,
Toronto, Ontario, Canada
[4]Department of Occupational Science & Occupational Therapy,
University of Toronto, Toronto, Ontario, Canada
[5]Early Childhood Studies, Ryerson University,
Toronto, Ontario, Canada

[*] Corresponding Author's E-mail: sukyoung.hong@mail.utoronto.ca.

## ABSTRACT

Children with autism spectrum disorder (ASD) often have fewer opportunities to participate in play than typically developing children because of their tendencies for repetitive play behaviours and preference for independent play. The Holland Bloorview (HB) *FIRST*® robotics program embeds technology into a playful activity that was designed to be accessible for children with disabilities. The objectives of the study included: (1) to measure pediatric volition among children with ASD participating in the robotics program, and (2) an exploratory objective to observe volitional behaviours among children with ASD in the robotics program. This study used a mixed-method design with a pediatric volitional questionnaire, video recordings and structured observations of 6 consecutive workshops. The results showed that pediatric volition had no statistically significant change in the total median score from the beginning to the end of the robotics program. However, through the observations children showed patterns of demonstrating interest and enjoyment of participating in the program.


**Keywords:** children, autism, play, robotics

## INTRODUCTION

Play is a critical component of a child's development that can help to foster self-determination, decision-making, and problem-solving skills (Lindsay & Lam, 2017). Exploring the development of play is important because limited play opportunities in early childhood can lead to social isolation and low self-esteem (Miller & Reid, 2003; Pollock et al., 1997). Children with disabilities often have fewer opportunities to engage in meaningful play compared to children without disabilities (Law et al., 2006; Lindsay & Lam, 2017). Exploring the development of play among children with autism spectrum disorder (ASD) is salient because they tend to engage in independent and repetitive play rather than playing with peers, in turn affecting the development of their social skills (Huijnen, Lexis, Jansens, & De Witte, 2016; Lindsay, Hounsell, & Cassiani, 2017). Therefore, providing an engaging environment that supports exploration, socialization, and learning may help children with disabilities to develop play skills (Lindsay & Lam, 2017). Although play is a vital way to motivate children, it is under-utilized as a therapeutic intervention (Couch, Deitz, & Kanny, 1998; Lindsay & Lam, 2017). As such, more research is needed to explore how play can be used as an intervention among children with disabilities (Lindsay & Lam, 2017). One promising play-based intervention is the Holland Bloorview (HB) *FIRST*® robotics program, which embeds technology into an accessible, playful activity (Lindsay & Hounsell, 2017).

Using robots as a form of play has the potential to increase children's development while also enhancing their interest in science, technology, engineering, and math (STEM) (Lindsay & Hounsell, 2017; Lindsay, Hounsell, & Cassiani, 2017). Developing STEM-related play through such mediums as LEGO® robotics is important for identifying children's volition (i.e., voluntary involvement in LEGO® robotics play) (Lindsay & Lam, 2017). Promoting STEM skills among children with disabilities is important because they tend to be significantly under-represented in STEM courses in school and in the workforce (Lindsay & Hounsell, 2017; Lindsay et al., 2017). Robotics interventions among youth without disabilities have shown that they have the potential to enhance motivation to explore STEM fields while also improving self-confidence, teamwork, collaboration, social, and communication skills (Benitti, 2012; Ludi & Reichlmayr, 2011). Many studies have proposed certain types of play or behavioral changes for children with disabilities, however, far fewer studies specifically target children with ASD. To date, only a few studies have explored the volition of children with ASD in a group-based LEGO® robotics play. According to previous studies, children with ASD often engage in more solitary play than collaborative play (Harper, Symon, & Frea, 2008; Libby, Weiss, Bancroft, & Ahearn, 2008; Lindsay & Lam, 2017). Even though children with ASD engage in solitary play, the majority of children with other types of disabilities often show signs of movement toward cooperative play through LEGO® robotics programs (Lindsay & Lam, 2017). Although children with ASD tend to engage less in collaborative or group-based play, exploring a group-based setting is salient because group-based play can promote diverse play skills and social skills, teamwork, and peer interaction in children with

ASD (Boyd et al., 2015; Harper et al., 2008; LeGoff, 2004; LeGoff & Sherman, 2006).

This study focused on children with ASD and their voluntary involvement in the HB *FIRST*® robotics program and how LEGO® robotics can contribute to the promotion of STEM skills among children with ASD. Although research in this area is growing, little is known about how an adapted robotics program can help to enhance play skills within the STEM-based activity among children with ASD.

# METHODS

## Objectives

The purpose of this research was to explore how children with ASD engage in play during a group-based adapted robotics program. The objectives of this study were: (1) To measure pediatric volition (i.e., the volitional behaviours demonstrated by each child during each robotics workshop) among children with ASD participating in an adapted robotics program (HB *FIRST*® robotics); and (2) to observe volitional behaviours among children with ASD in the robotics program.

## Mixed-Methods Design

This research drew on data from a larger study by Lindsay et al. (2017; 2019) that focused on the impact of the HB FIRST® robotics program. In this current study we used a mixed-methods design with pre- and post-score comparison, and video-recorded, structured observations of each robotics workshop (Lindsay & Hounsell, 2017; Lindsay et al., 2017). The mixed methods design (Bradt, Burns, & Creswell, 2013) was chosen to provide in-depth understanding of children's volitional behavior observed in an adapted robotics program (Bradt et al., 2013).

The embedded design involves four phases: 1) concurrent collection of quantitative and qualitative data; 2) primary emphasis given to quantitative data; 3) separate analysis of quantitative and qualitative data; and 4) integration and mixing of the two data sets at the level of data interpretation (Creswell, Plano Clark, Gutmann, & Hanson, 2003).

## Sample and Recruitment

The study drew from a larger investigation exploring the impact of an adapted robotics program on play and STEM skills among children with disabilities (Lindsay et al. 2019). For this study, we focused on one level of the program (i.e., junior level I) because they had high number of youth with ASD to explore. All youth who took part in two groups of the junior level I, HB *FIRST*® robotics program were eligible to participate and received an information package and consent form from the researcher. Children and their parent signed a written consent/assent form, and the researcher asked if they had any questions prior to engaging in the study. Ethics approval was obtained from the Bloorview Research Institute Research Ethics Board (REB) and the University of Toronto REB prior to starting the study.

## Inclusion Criteria

Inclusion criteria for this HB *FIRST*® robotics program included the following: (a) Youth with a disability, (b) clients of a pediatric rehabilitation center, (c) aged 6-10 (d) expressed an interest LEGO® or robotics and/or who may benefit from the workshop, and (e) parents were supportive of youth's participation in the workshop. For this study, only those with ASD were included in the analysis.

## Procedure

The HB *FIRST*® robotics program is an adapted version of *FIRST*® robotics Canada (Lindsay & Hounsell, 2017; Lindsay et al., 2019). This program engaged children in designing, building, and programming robots to solve everyday problems (Lindsay & Hounsell, 2017). Children built models that reflected each week's lesson, where they learned things such as simple machines (i.e., gears, pulleys, levers, and sensors) using the LEGO® WeDo® software, and then created a program to show its movement, connecting their completed robots to an iPad.

For this study, we focussed on one age-group: junior level I (aged 6-10 years) (Lindsay et al. 2019). Level I was designed to learn basic concepts of coding and robots whereas level II (reported elsewhere) is designed to learn advanced concept of coding and robots (Lindsay et al., 2019). The program involved six consecutive workshops (two hours each, once a week) where children learned to design and build LEGO® robotics models; explore challenges facing today's scientists; engage in team activities; and participate in a celebration event (Lindsay et al., 2019). Each child had a partner and a skilled adult volunteer and/or a therapist (e.g., therapeutic recreation specialist) that helped them build their robot (Lindsay & Hounsell, 2017). Each workshop had a new learning objective and challenge, and each youth took turns being the builder and the engineer (i.e., the person who finds the right piece to connect LEGO® blocks). Through each week's learning objectives, children learned different concepts (i.e., pull-robot with concept of pulleys; helicopter with concept of gears; garbage truck with concept of math and distance) (Lindsay et al., 2019).

Each workshop began with a 20-minute "build to express" activity allowing children to build something with the LEGO® pieces of their own interest, while listening to others, sharing, and learning (Lindsay et al., 2019). Next, children had an opportunity to watch a short video on an iPad, highlighting some challenges facing today's scientists. Then, children had the opportunity to build and test the robot themselves while working with a partner (Lindsay et al., 2019). Children were paired, alternating between being the builder and the designer (Lindsay & Hounsell, 2017; 2019). The designer was responsible for conveying information to their partner on how to assemble the robot, and the builder put the pieces together (Lindsay & Hounsell, 2017). A challenge was then posed to the groups (i.e., move completed robots in different directions, or code different sounds). In the last 15 minutes of each workshop parents were invited into the room to see what the children had made (Lindsay et al., 2019).

## Data Collection

Data were collected from two separate groups (group 1: October 4 to November 8, 2017; group 2: January 24 to February 28, 2018). Even though there were two different groups occurring at different times, they learned the same concepts each workshop. Therefore, we combined the two groups (i.e., group 1 and group 2) in the analysis process rather than analyzing them separately. Quantitative data were collected from only Time 1 (the first workshop) and Time 2 (the fifth workshop) to compare changes between the beginning of the program and the last of the program. Qualitative data (i.e., observations) were collected from all workshops (i.e., from the first workshop to the fifth workshop). Even though the program involved six workshops for each group, the current study used the fifth workshop for Time 2 because the sixth week was a celebration event and did not involve learning new concepts. The program took place in a classroom at a children's hospital. Each classroom had five volunteers with experience in robotics, plus one therapeutic recreation specialist, and a robotics education coordinator (Lindsay et al., 2019).

The following measures were used to assess play skills among youth with ASD: pediatric volitional questionnaires and HB *FIRST*® robotics observational template. Demographic information were also collected through a survey distributed to participants' parents prior to starting the program.

## Primary Outcome: Pediatric Volitional Questionnaires (PVQ)

The Pediatric Volitional Questionnaire (PVQ) was designed to capture a child's inner motivations and information about how the environment or activity relates to the child's volition (Harris & Reid, 2005). This measure was developed in response to a need for assessing the volition that was appropriate for children (Andersen et al., 2005; Liu et al., 2013). It examines a child's volitional behavior in an environment or activities, using a 14-item, 4-point rating scale designed for observation of children ages 2-7, yielding a measurement of volition (Andersen et al., 2005; Harris & Reid, 2005; Miller et al., 2014). The 14 behavioral indicators of volition are distributed along a continuum of volitional proceeding from three sub-categories: 1) exploration (i.e., the client desires to engage in the environment for pleasure and enjoyment, and to make discoveries in low risk situations); to 2) competence (i.e., the client has a drive to actively interact with and influence the environment, practice skills, and meet performance standards); and 3) achievement (i.e., the client strives to increase their capacity to do a challenging task and to have successful performance outcomes) (Andersen et al., 2005; Harris & Reid, 2005; Miller, Ziviani, Ware, & Boyd, 2016).

The scoring system for the PVQ involves a 4-point rating scale including the following: 0 (N/A), 1 (passive), 2 (hesitant), 3 (involved), 4 (spontaneous), enabling the client to demonstrate volitional behavior (Andersen et al., 2005). The highest score is 4 (spontaneous) and indicates that the child must have shown the behaviours without support, structure, or encouragement, while 1 (passive) indicates the child did not demonstrate the behavior, even with support, structure, or encouragement (Andersen et al., 2005). With the scoring system, the highest total score is 56 (Andersen et al., 2005; Liu et al., 2013). In addition to measuring volition, the PVQ was also designed to observe qualitative information about volitionally related environment and activities (Andersen et al., 2005). The PVQ has good construct validity in capturing volition (Andersen et al., 2005; Harris & Reid, 2005; Liu et al., 2013; Miller et al., 2014). It is a valid measure of volition that is well evidenced in the literature (Andersen et al., 2005; Liu et al., 2013).

## Inter-Rater Reliability

To ensure inter-rater reliability, PVQ scoring was scored independently by two different people (first author and a research assistant) who were trained in using the measures. We independently reviewed 28 videos and then scored the PVQ. After coding the videos and scoring separately each of our scores were compared. Both raters met and discussed scores and any discrepancies. There were less than 5 discrepancies per scoring. When there were wide discrepancies in certain items, the raters discussed or re-watched the videos to narrow any discrepancies until agreement was reached. Given that the percent of agreement as a measure of inter-rater reliability, did not consider random agreements (Fischer & Neumann, 2012), we used Cohen's kappa to assess inter-rater reliability in this study (Fischer & Neumann, 2012; McHugh, 2012). We entered all PVQ scores into SPSS, and Cohen's kappa values for PVQ were 0.82 (almost perfect agreement) (Cohen, 1960).

## Exploratory Outcome: Observations

We used the HB *FIRST*® robotics observation (i.e., project-specific) template (Lindsay and Hounsell, 2017) to assess verbal and non-verbal behaviours that signal the child's behaviours. This template involves 4 parts: enabling observers to capture children's behavior in different stages (e.g., build to express, sharing, deciding roles, and activity) (see Lindsay and Hounsell, 2017). Observers wrote down their observations while participants built each week's LEGO® model.

## Data Analysis

In this study, two sets of data (quantitative and qualitative) were combined and mixed at the stage of results and interpretation. Quantitative findings (e.g., Wilcoxon signed-rank test) was used, whereas, qualitative findings (e.g., observation notes from the HB *FIRST*® robotics template) were used to enhance and support quantitative findings.

## Quantitative Data

Quantitative data involved PVQ scores, which we entered into SPSS, version 25. Means, standard deviations, medians, and ranges addressed the main objective of the study. We performed a non-parametric test due to skewness in the data (Corrado, 1989; Fagerland, 2012; Groenveld & Meeden, 1984). As the equivalent non-parametric test for the paired sample t-test is the paired samples Wilcoxon test, the Wilcoxon signed-rank test was conducted (Corrado, 1989; Fagerland, 2012; Groeneveld & Meeden, 1984; Rey & Neuhäuser, 2011). Skewness, mean, standard deviation, median, and range were analyzed to answer the quantitative objective (i.e., to measure pediatric volition among children with ASD participating in an adapted robotics program) using an alpha of 0.05. Participants' demographic data (e.g., age, disability type, participation) were reviewed to assess whether it may have affected the results of the study.

For the main objective outcome, median scores of PVQ were analyzed to understand children's pediatric volition. We collected PVQ scores from 5 weeks for each group. We did not assess the 6$^{th}$ week because they did not build a model but rather it was a celebration event. These scores were analyzed and plotted on graphs. The first author and a research assistant independently completed the PVQ scoring for each participant at the end of each workshop. Each workshop was also video-recorded, to enable the researchers to explore observations in further in-depth and to verify agreement in the scores.

## Qualitative Data

For the exploratory outcome, the qualitative data consisted of notes from the observation template and recorded videos which were analyzed to verify the content of the observations. This study used a conventional content analysis approach (Hsieh & Shannon, 2005) and a constructionism paradigm to answer the exploratory objective and to understand the qualitative data (Atieno, 2009; Elo & Kyngäs, 2008; Hunt, 2009). The philosophical assumption from constructionism in the study helped to explain the quantitative outcomes in greater depth as two observers analyzed and interpreted the qualitative data (i.e., observation notes) in a subjective manner (Creswell, Shope, Plano Clark, & Green, 2006; Hsieh & Shannon, 2005; Vaismoradi, Jones, Turunen, & Snelgrove, 2016).

The two observers, trained in qualitative observations, independently collected observation notes according to the four different sections for each participant during each workshop of the robotics program. Even though the observation notes were collected from workshop 1 to workshop 6, analysis of observation notes focused only on time 1 and time 2. The first author coded and categorized all observation notes line-by-line (Graneheim & Lundman, 2004; Hsieh & Shannon, 2005). Two authors read the full observation text several times before coding and categorizing, to obtain a full sense of the whole dataset (Graneheim & Lundman, 2004; Hsieh & Shannon, 2005). We extracted relevant behaviours or noted examples based on the words or observational contents such as 'stays focused', 'stays in participation', 'tries to solve problems', and any related similar content of notes (e.g., seems focused, participates well, shows teamwork, joins others, expresses pride in accomplishment) under "volitional behaviours" (Anderson, Kielhofner, & Lai, 2005; Lindsay, McPherson, & Maxwell, 2017). Keywords of observations were generated based on reviews of the literature on either pediatric volitional questionnaire (Anderson, Kielhofner, & Lai, 2005). We then synthesized and read extracted examples several times to ensure the observation examples were comprehensive and captured relevant observation notes to volitional behaviours (Graneheim & Lundman, 2004). Following the research questions, any observational content related to volitional behaviors were coded and categorized (Hsieh & Shannon, 2005).

Two observers met and to discuss the categorization of the content (Hsieh & Shannon, 2005; Vaismoradi et al., 2016). The second observer checked the coded and categorized content (Fischer & Neumann, 2012). Where there was any disagreement, the two observers discussed until there was consensus of an optimal fit between the observation and the categories (Fischer & Neumann, 2012). Any observations that were in disagreement were discussed and revised (Fischer & Neumann, 2012). Discussion between the two observers and the research team led to the identification of patterns and themes (Graneheim & Lundman, 2004).

## Rigour and Trustworthiness

We applied several strategies to ensure the rigor and credibility of the observation outcomes (e.g., truth value, consistency, applicability) (Krefting, 1991; Noble & Smith, 2015). A 'truth value' is used as an indicator of 'validity' in qualitative research. We outlined participants' playful experiences during the robotics program, to ensure the truth value of qualitative data (Noble & Smith, 2015). 'Consistency' was used as an indicator of 'reliability' in the current research (Noble & Smith, 2015). For consistency and reliability, the content analysis included member checking (i.e., verification and discussions) amongst the observers involved in the robotics program who watched the videos then observed and collected data throughout the six-week adapted robotics program. Two observers re-watched the videos if there were disagreements and discussed until both agreed on the content. In addition, we used descriptive quotes from the observation notes. Even though our experience may have influenced our interpretation of the analysis, the two observers both agreed on the content of observation for data verification (Hunt, 2009). Finally, we assessed 'applicability' and 'generalisability' (Noble & Smith, 2015). The qualitative observations itself included valid experiences of participants and these were verified by the observers. Therefore, through valid and reliable data collection, the study can be considered applicable to other contexts or groups (Krefting, 1991; Noble & Smith, 2015).

# RESULTS

In total, 14 children with ASD participated in an adapted HB *FIRST*® robotics program (see Table 1). All participants were male and had ASD. Three of them had more than one condition (i.e., ADHD, intellectual disability, or learning disability) (see Table 1). Their ages ranged from 6 to 10 and the mean age was 7.79.

**Table 1. Overview of participant characteristics**

| **Demographic** | **Group 1** | **Group 2** |
|---|---|---|
| Workshops | 6 workshops | 6 workshops |
| Gender | Male | Male |
| Number of Participants | 7 | 7 |
| Disability | 4 ASD<br>1 ASD and ADHD<br>1 ASD and Intellectual Disability<br>1 ASD and learning disability | 7 ASD |
| Age | 6-9 (mean age: 7.43) | 6-10 (mean age: 8.14) |
| Number of workshops attended mean (SD) | 5.29 (0.95) | 6.00 (0.00) |
| Number of times shared mean (SD) | 4.29 (0.95) | 4.29 (1.11) |
| Partnered with | 6 (with peer)<br>1 (with adult volunteer) | 5 (with peer)<br>2 (with adult volunteer) |
| Participated in the program before | First time: 11 participants (78.6%) | |
| | Second time: 2 participants (14.3%) | |
| | Fourth time: 1 participant (7.1%) | |
| Participation for 6 weeks | 4 times: 1 (7.1%) | |
| | 5 times: 2 (14.3%) | |
| | All 6 times: 11 (78.8%) | |

The majority of participants (78.6%) took part in the HB *FIRST*® robotics program for the first time (see Table 1). Among the total of 14 participants, two had participated one time previously, and one had participated four times in the same level and the same program. The majority of children (78.8%) participated all six workshops, whereas, two participants

(14.3%) missed one class, and one (7.1%) missed two classes of the six-week program. Twelve children (85.7%) shared their model in front of the class at time 1, meanwhile 13 children (92.9%) shared their model in time 2. One child never shared on his own LEGO® model during any of the workshops, despite encouragement from staff.

## Pediatric Volition Questionnaire

The statistics indicated that there was a subtle mean change in PVQ total score from Time 1 ($M$ = 41.00, $SD$ = 12.18) to Time 2 ($M$ = 39.07, $SD$ = 9.20). The mean decrease in PVQ total mean was 1.93, with a 95% confident interval ranging from -5.23 to 9.09. Even though there was a subtle decrease in PVQ total mean, the Wilcoxon signed-rank test indicated that there was no statistically significant change in PVQ total score from Time 1 ($Mdn$ = 45.00) to Time 2 ($Mdn$ = 42.00), $Z = -0.28$, $p = 0.780$ (two-tailed) (see Figure 1 and Table 2).

## Qualitative Results

The outcome of qualitative results were to answer exploratory objective in the current study. The findings resulted in one main theme (i.e., the participants explored in the HB *FIRST*® robotics program) and one sub-theme (i.e., participants showed involvement in the given tasks). The results are organized according to the four components of the program (i.e., build to express, sharing, teaching, LEGO® activity), during the HB *FIRST*® robotics program.

Fourteen participants displayed similar patterns of volitional behaviour in the sub-theme (i.e., they showed involvement in the program). We first describe the flow of the four components of the program, then the sub-theme was expressed during the program: involvement in the program.

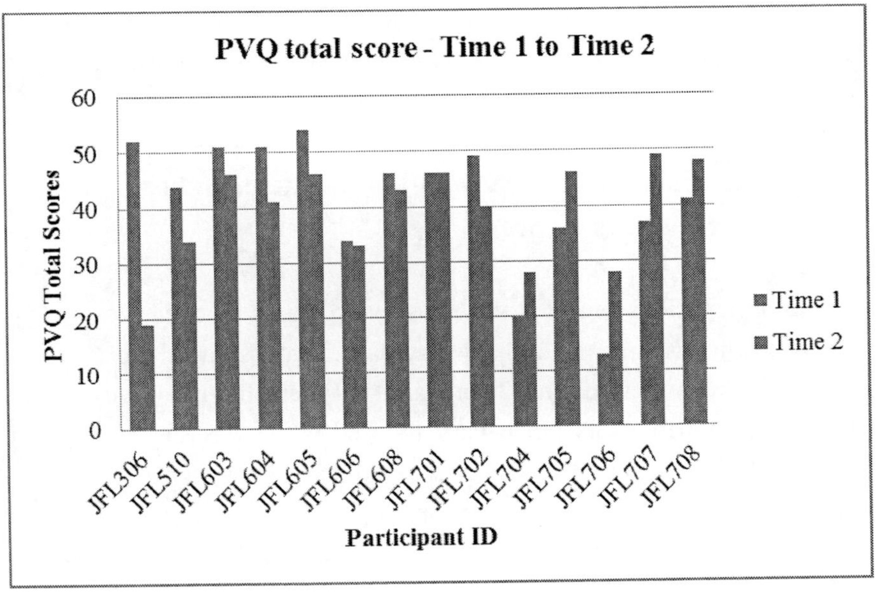


Figure 1. PVQ Total Scores from Time 1 to Time 2.

**Table 2. Wilcoxon Signed-Rank Test for Pediatric Volition Questionnaire (PVQ)**

| | | **Mean** | ***SD*** | **Range** | **Median** | **Z** | **Sig. (2-tailed)** |
|---|---|---|---|---|---|---|---|
| PVQ Score | **Total** PVQ Time1 | 41.00 | 12.18 | 41 | 45.00 | - 0.28 | 0.780 |
| | **Total** PVQ Time2 | 39.07 | 9.20 | 30 | 42.00 | | |

### *Theme and Sub-Theme*

The main theme comprises one sub-theme. The sub-theme is described below with supporting examples from participants. Participants experienced patterns of showing volitional behaviours during the robotics program, which included: being involved in the given tasks; willing to participate in the activities; seeming focused; and related similar observational content (e.g., seemed interested, participated actively, modelled teamwork).

Participants showed patterns of willingness to participate in the activities and seemed focused, satisfied in their work and interested at time 2.

## Sub-Theme: Participants Showed Involvement in the Given Tasks Build to Express

The observations revealed that most participants enjoyed the 'build to express' portion (i.e., free-play). Twelve participants showed more patterns of volitional behaviours at time 2 compared to time 1. In time 1, we observed that participant JFL702 seemed very focused while creating his LEGO® model, and participant JFL707 clapped, talked and showed off his LEGO® model to volunteers and therapists with a happy voice (observer 1, time 1). However, participant JFL306 preferred to partner with adult volunteers rather than with peer partners (observer 1, time 1). Compared to time 1, participants showed more examples of volitional behaviours in time 2. Twelve of 14 participants seemed to enjoy LEGO® building during 'build to express' (observers 1 and 2, time 2). In addition, participant JFL705 seemed proud of his own LEGO® model (observer 1, time 2), and participant JFL702 seemed very interested during 'build to express', staying focused on what he was doing while his peer partner showed less interest in the activity (observer 1, time 2).

## Sharing

Two participants showed notable volitional behaviours in the sharing portion of the program in time 1. For example, participants JFL604 and JFL705 voluntarily raised their hands to share LEGO® models, and they explained in detail their LEGO® models in front of the class (observer 1, time 1). On the other hand, at time 2, 13 children shared their LEGO® models in front of the class, and the children's sharing skills were confident and full of vivid descriptions. For example, we observed that participant JFL608 showed confidence when sharing his LEGO® models, and his description included vivid, imaginative descriptions. His voice was full of confidence and his presentation skill was excellent (observer 1, time 2). In addition, participant JFL705 faced the audience when presenting his LEGO® models, and his descriptions were full of detailed explanations. Participant JFL705 also showed great skill in asking questions. He asked many questions about his peers' LEGO® models, using appropriate manners, such as, 'What is that next to that?' 'I really like your model,' or 'That's so cool!' (observer 1, time 2).

A few children were eager to raise their hands to share their model and exhibited great skill in describing their LEGO® models but not in answering questions. Participant JFL604 always raised his hand and was eager to share his LEGO® model, though he did not complete the LEGO® creation (observer 1, time 2). Participant JFL603 also liked sharing his LEGO® model and showed volitional behaviour, such as raising his hand and presenting in front of the class; but he did not make eye contact with a therapist or peers when they asked questions (observer 1, time 2).

Meanwhile, not all children liked and enjoyed the 'sharing' portion of the class. For instance, participants JFL606 and JFL704 did not raise their hands to share their LEGO® models. Adult volunteers prompted them to participate and encouraged them to share their LEGO® creations. When they stood up in front of the class at a volunteer's prompting, participants did not start to talk by themselves. Instead, the program coordinator or volunteer asked presenters questions such as, 'What is this?' and 'Why did you make this?' Then participants JFL606 and JFL704 answered with a word or an incomplete sentence, such as 'tree' or 'standing building' (observer 1, times 1 and 2).

## Teaching

In the teaching portion, there were no notable observational changes in volitional behaviours from time 1 to time 2. Children freely raised their hands to share their thoughts and opinions on learning new topics. Participant JFL306, for example, seemed very interested in each week's topic, but he did not like all the topics. He had already participated four times in this same level and of the program. Sometimes it seemed he had already learned the same concept previously, and so he seemed less focused and interested in the topics he had already experienced. When he already knew about the topic, participant JFL306 tried to play a video clip on an iPad while the robotic coordinator was talking. The volunteers needed to prompt him to turn off the iPad and listen to the robotic coordinator's instruction (observer 1, times 1 and 2). Another participant, JFL605, seemed very interested in each week's topic and he showed volitional behaviour such as asking questions regarding the topic (observer 1, time 2). In addition, all participants seemed to enjoy watching the short LEGO® video clip on an iPad. We observed that most children were focused while watching the clip, in times 1 and 2.

## LEGO® Robotics Activity

In the LEGO® robotics building portion, volitional behaviours such as seeming focused and interested, completing the activity by oneself, modelling good teamwork, and cooperating well were observed more in time 2. Observers found that children were eager to build and assemble LEGO® robots and enjoyed working with partners. Some examples from observations: participant JFL306 worked well and seemed focused on assembling LEGO® blocks. He seemed very interested and eager to build LEGO® robots (observer 2, time 1). Participants JFL604 and JFL605 also seemed interested in LEGO® activities. They mostly assembled and completed LEGO® robots by themselves (observers 1 and 2, time 1).

We observed that participant JFL701 exhibited good teamwork with his peer partner. He often asked questions of his peer partner if he was not sure about the next steps. In addition, JFL701 and his peer partner had discussions when they faced difficult parts during the activity. Participant JFL701 often built and connected LEGO® in sequence by himself (observer 1, time 2). In another example, we found that participant JFL702 modelled good teamwork with his peer partner. He tried to connect LEGO® blocks step by step, asking for help after trying first but having a hard time finding the right place to connect the LEGO® pieces (observer 1, times 1 and 2). In another instance, we noted that JFL510 continued to focus on building LEGO®. Sometimes volunteers gave him hints to complete the LEGO® assembly steps, and then he enjoyed completing LEGO® robots (observer 1, time 2). Participant JFL702 showed high focus on what he was doing, even though his peer partner did not participate well. When his peer partner did not pass him LEGO® blocks, JFL702 demonstrated how to find the right LEGO® piece, and he completed the LEGO® robot (observer 1, time 2).

We also observed a few touching moments of how children enjoyed the activity and were proud of themselves. Participant JFL705 showed his LEGO® robot to his dad, saying proudly, 'Dad, look what I did! This part can move this way and I programmed it! Cool!' (observer 1, time 2). Participant JFL606 picked up his LEGO® robot and said enthusiastically to his mom, 'Mom, look this. I made this. Don't you so proud of me? I am so proud of myself. This is the robot that I made for the first time!' His mother looked at him with a smile and hugged him (observer 1, time 2).

## Discussion

The objective of the study was to explore the pediatric volition among children with ASD participating in the HB *FIRST*® robotics program. For the main objective, children aged 6–10 with ASD were expected to achieve pediatric volitional scores significantly higher than their baseline scores in play after participating in the HB *FIRST*® robotics program. However, participants in this study did not show a statistically significant increase in pediatric volition scores. The second (exploratory) objective observed the volitional behaviours among children with ASD during an adapted robotics program. Despite the non-significant PVQ statistical results, the observation notes revealed patterns of willingness to participate and interest in the activities.

## Pediatric Volition in an Adapted Robotics Play

There were no significant results from the quantitative findings, though there were several encouraging observations of volitional behaviour. The favorable volitional behavior demonstrated among the participants included: staying involved with given tasks, willingness to participate in activities, remaining focused, being satisfied with work results, cooperating with turn-taking during LEGO® building, engaging in problem-solving, and expressing interest and enjoyment in activities. Although previous studies show that an adapted robotics program can improve interest in Science, Technology, Engineering, and Mathematics (STEM) skills among children with disabilities (Cheng et al., 2013; Lamptey et al., 2019; Lindsay & Hounsell, 2017; Lindsay et al., 2017; Lindsay & Lam, 2017), results of the current study were partially consistent with these previous studies. The quantitative findings were inconsistent with previous studies, whereas subtheme one from the qualitative findings revealed that the participants showed more cases of positive volitional behaviour that confirmed that an adapted robotics program can be worthwhile and enjoyable for children with disabilities (Lamptey et al., 2019; Lindsay & Hounsell, 2017; Lindsay et al., in review). One potential reason for the current study's quantitative findings on PVQ being contradictory to those of previous studies could be due to the small sample size (Lindsay et al., 2017; Lindsay et al., 2019). Non-significant findings for pediatric volition over the course of the program could be attributed to the following: 1) the sample size (n = 14) was small; 2) three of the participants were repeating the same program; 3) results cannot be generalized because there were no female participants; and 4) not all of the children may have benefited from one-to-one support from an adult volunteer. In addition, the children could not choose their own partners, and it is possible that those who were not satisfied with their assigned partner may have shown decreased PVQ.

## Reduction in PVQ

Although the results of the qualitative findings of the current study were meaningful and encouraging, the statistical findings were not significant, perhaps because the sample size was not large enough to detect a significant difference (Creswell, 2014; Lamptey et al., 2019). In addition, a number of elements may have restricted an increase in pediatric volition. First, children who previously participated in the same program may have felt a lower level of interest in the repetition of the same LEGO® play. The repetition of the LEGO® play may have resulted in decreasing PVQ scores of the current study. However, the current study was inconsistent with results from previous study. For example, Therrien, Wickstrom, and Jones (2006) conducted a study investigating how a repeated intervention improves the reading achievement of students with learning disabilities (Therrien et al., 2006). Participants in that study included fourth-to-eighth grades students, with a learning disability in reading or at risk of reading failure (Therrien et al., 2006). The students were assigned to either a treatment or control group via stratified random assignment (Therrien et al., 2006). Students in the treatment group received a repeated reading intervention. The study confirmed that the repeated reading intervention significantly improved the treatment group's reading speed of passages, comprehension, and oral reading fluency (Therrien et al., 2006). Although the type of interventions for the reading and the current LEGO® robotics study were different, the research design of repetition was parallel (Terrien et al., 2006). While the previous study confirmed that repeated intervention can improve a certain performance, the current study did not indicate a positive effect from repeated intervention. Repeating participants in the current study seemed to demonstrate less interest in concepts they had already learned or experienced by building the same LEGO® robots. Repeated interventions may improve performance skills but could also decrease interest. In the current study, decreased pediatric volition scores and observation notes both suggested that repeated participants showed decreased interest in the same LEGO® activity. Decreased interest may be connected to lower volition, as volition refers to voluntarily performing of an action. Therefore, participants' interest may decrease through a repeated intervention, in turn resulting in decreased volition while completing the same LEGO® activity.

Additionally, the current study involved only male participants. Research examining pediatric volition among girls with disabilities in a group-based robotics program (Lindsay et al., 2019) found a significant increase in the participants' pediatric volition scores from the beginning to the end of the program. The findings of the current study, however, are inconsistent with those results. Although the current program was open to all genders, no females enrolled in the program during the period of recruitment for this study. However, the study by Kolne and Lindsay (2019) was partially consistent with the current study and it may give a potential avenue for the current study. Kolne and Lindsay (2019) explored the interaction between teachers and children with disabilities (18 with ASD, 3 with CP, and 1 with Duchenne muscular dystrophy) enrolled in an adapted robotics program to examine potential gender differences. 8 girls and 14 boys were participated in the study (Kolne & Lindsay, 2019). Overall, children in the all-boys program indicated a more passive engagement (i.e., primarily speak only when prompted and indirect response to a teacher's question) during robotics instruction, whereas, children in the all-girls program indicated a more active engagement (i.e., speak more without being prompted by the teacher and ask more questions) with the teachers during the instruction (Kolne & Lindsay, 2019). As proposed from previous studies (Kolne & Lindsay, 2019; Lindsay et al., 2019), children in all-girls program indicated a more active engagement and showed significant pediatric volitional improvements. Therefore, participants' gender may have influence in the current findings.

In another related study, Harrop et al. (2017) conducted a study to examine the play complexity of girls and boys with ASD, in comparison to typically developing girls and boys. They found no significant differences in play complexity or toy engagement between preschool-age girls and boys with ASD (Harrop et al., 2017). Both ASD and typically developing girls, however, were more engaged in playing with dolls and domestic items (e.g., food items, utensils, shopping baskets) than boys with ASD or without disabilities (Harrop et al., 2017). Boys with ASD, on the other hand, engaged with toys such as a garage and cars for a longer time than girls with ASD (Harrop et al., 2017). Although the girls and boys engaged for different lengths of time with a variety of types of toys, the study suggested that girls with ASD may engage in similar types of play as boys with ASD (Harrop et al., 2017). In the current study, the HB FIRST® robotics coordinator chose each week's topic and types of LEGO® robots (e.g., garbage truck, rescue helicopter). Although the program was the same but with different choices of LEGO® robots, girls with disabilities showed a significant increase in pediatric volition (Lindsay et al., 2019), while the boys in the current study did not show a significant increase in volition. Harrop et al. (2017) claimed that boys and girls may engage for different lengths of time with different types of toys, and the choice of LEGO® robots may therefore affect volitional changes. Girls in the same program showed a significant increase in their volitional score, perhaps because they liked the choice of the LEGO® robots. Meanwhile, the boys in the current study showed decreased volitional scores, perhaps because they did not like the choice of LEGO® robots. Therefore, the gender of the participants in the current study may have influenced the results, and the choice of LEGO® robots may have decreased the male participants' volitional scores. However, further research is required to assess this observation in further depth.

This study did not examine how individual variation, such as choice of peer partner, play familiarity, or personality, affected the PVQ among children with ASD (Alagendran, Hitch, Wadley, & Stagnitti, 2019). Askins et al. (2013) investigated the intrinsic motivation among children with developmental disabilities which was measured using the PVQ. Their study found that most children demonstrated increased pediatric volitional behaviour: spontaneously showing preferences, trying to produce effects, demonstrating curiosity, and expressing mastery pleasure in their natural environment (Askins, Diasio, Szewerniak, & Cahill, 2013). Even though the study by Askins et al. (2013) used the same measurement as the current study, the study did not compare PVQ scores between the two time points (Time 1 and Time 2). However, Askins et al. (2013) suggested that a child's unique needs should be considered during a play activity (Askins et al., 2013). In the current study, the children did not choose their peer partner or adult volunteer. Even though the children could change their peer partner each week, it was difficult to determine whether a match was a positive one. Considering each child's unique needs, a partner match may affect a child's volitional changes. Although the current study offered opportunities to experience LEGO® robotics activities with peers, an unwelcomed peer-match could influence volitional behavioral change among children with ASD.

The current study showed no significant improvement in volition through PVQ measurement. One of the reasons of non-significant findings was non-supportive one-to-one support from adult volunteers and partner choices. Although the study by Salter, Beamish, and Davies (2016) did not use the same measurement, it suggested possible improvement concerning positive reciprocal interaction and environment. Salter, Beamish, and Davies (2016) conducted research to explore the effects of child-centered play therapy (CCPT) on the social and emotional growth of three young Australian children with autism, aged 4 to 6 years (Salter, Beamish & Davies, 2016). They used two measurements: the Adaptive Behaviour Assessment System, Second Edition, Parent Form (ABAS-II) and the Developmental Behaviour Checklist-Parent/Care giver (DBC-P) within pre- and post-intervention (Salter, Beamish & Davies, 2016) design. The CCPT intervention was undertaken over 10 weeks, and each child attended 50 minute sessions with the same trained therapist (Salter, Beamish & Davies, 2016). As a result, ABAS-II and DBC-P indicated that all children improved in several areas of social and emotional functioning and progressed in the targeted goal areas which were identified by parents (Salter, Beamish & Davies, 2016). Their overall findings were consistent with previous literature showing each CCPT intervention was effective in assisting participating children to enhance their social and emotional skills (Salter, Beamish & Davies, 2016). In the current study, I noted that not every child may have benefited from one-to-one support from adult volunteers. As Salter, Beamish and Davies (2016) proposed, a positive reciprocal interaction with therapists and the environment may foster enhancement of social skills, emotional skills, and targeted problem areas among children with ASD (Salter, Beamish & Davies, 2016). Therefore, the quantitative results in volition might not have shown meaningful improvement among children with ASD in the current study, because the study did not control a complete supportive play environment through adult volunteers or partners.

## Positive Patterns in Volitional Behaviour

Although the current study did not assess STEM experiences, previous research may be consistent in showing positive behavioural improvements after participating in the HB FIRST® robotics program. Previous research focusing on a robotics program for children with disabilities showed that it can be helpful with learning computer programming and fostering an interest in science, technology, engineering, and mathematics (STEM) (Lindsay & Hounsell, 2017). The results of a study by Lindsay and Hounsell (2017) highlighted that a robotics program might be an important mechanism for developing potential career interests of youth with disabilities (Lindsay & Hounsell, 2017). In the current study, I observed that most children enjoyed connecting LEGO® blocks and were pleased when they could code and program their own LEGO® robots. Though the current study did not assess whether the HB FIRST® robotics program might be an important mechanism for developing potential career interest in children with disabilities, the study's qualitative findings indicated that the robotics program described pediatric volition among children with ASD, and that participants demonstrated interest, satisfaction and involvement in the given activities.

The current study also observed signs of volitional behaviour in the HB FIRST® robotics program. LeGoff and Sherman (2006) additionally conducted research on interactive LEGO® play to investigate long-term outcomes of social skills. Their study comprised both individual and group sessions continuously over three years (Legoff & Sherman, 2006). The study used measurements such as the Vinland Adaptive Behaviour socialization domain (VABS-SD) and GARS social interaction (GARS-SI) scale to assess social competence and social skills rather than pediatric volition (Legoff & Sherman, 2006). It was determined that LEGO® play participants showed great improvement in a broad range of social skills and a reduction in autistic-type social behaviors compared to their matched control (Legoff & Sherman, 2006). Although the current thesis did not aim to investigate children's social skills, the observation notes in the study include a few positive signs of social skill improvement: participants completed their tasks, asked for assistance in an appropriate manner, peer partner teamwork improved, and participants shared their LEGO® robots in front of the class with descriptive explanations. Therefore, although the current study did not investigate the children's social skills, findings indicate the activity's potential for children's social skill improvement. Future research should be conducted to explore the role of adult behavior and interaction with the children to assess the impact this may have had on their motivation and participation in the program.

Additionally, Peplak et al. investigated how children reason their inclusion decisions in the context of play (Peplak, Song, Colasante, & Malti, 2017). Their results showed that the majority of children decided to include play members regardless of age and context, but children preferred to include peers who do not display negative behaviour, such as not paying attention during play or pushing another child (Peplak et al., 2017). The study suggested that children often want to include peers who promote a play goal, and exclude peers who may threaten them or cast a negative light on their image (Peplak et al., 2017). Building on previous literature, the current study also provided opportunities to explore pediatric volition in a group-based setting in which children had opportunities to explore their play with peers. Children in the current study, however, were unable to choose their own partners. Children with ASD often encounter difficulty with play behaviors and peer interaction because of their repetitive play behaviour and more independent play repertories, compared to typically developing peers (Alagendran et al., 2019; Godin et al., 2017; Lee et al., 2017). Lindsay and Lam (2017), for example, investigated the types of play children engage in while taking part in a LEGO® robotics program. Their results showed that the adapted LEGO® robotics program provided opportunities to develop play skills and rapport with peers (Lindsay & Lam, 2017). The current study with the HB FIRST® robotics program itself might provide opportunities to develop play skills with peers, but undesired matches may have influenced change in volitional behavioral.

### Future Directions

Future research should be directed to several areas. Further studies should explore potential play skills and types by different disability types. Different level of assistance, level of play, and familiarity of context are all potential areas to improve the current study. Second, more research is needed to explore gender differences in pediatric volition among children with ASD. As there were only boys in our study, it would be important to include girls and investigate gender differences in pediatric volition. Third, researchers and clinicians should consider the longer-term impact from robotics programs on pediatric volition outcomes.

Future research could involve children with more disability types, with a range of needs and skills, and more varied play types such as solitary play and parallel play (Lindsay & Lam, 2017). Offering different levels of play activities (i.e., easy, medium, hard) according to children's cognition levels, could offer children benefits from greater play vocabulary and more extensive play repertoire, such as different play types, unexpected utterances, and suggestions. If, for example, the intervention has different levels of programming, then children with different cognition and learning levels could choose the most appropriate program. Finally, future studies should consider and explore factors (e.g., partnership, repeated participation) in increasing or decreasing children's PVQ.

## Conclusion

Play is an essential component of children's development and our study explored pediatric volition among children with autism in a robotics program. Although there was no significant improvement in pediatric volition scores, there were positive patterns of volitional behaviour through observation. Further research is needed to understand the longer-term impacts of the robotics program.

## ACKNOWLEDGMENTS

We would like to thank the staff and students in the TRAIL lab in the Bloorview Research Institute who contrubited to this project. The first author received a MSc scholarhship from the Social Science and Humanities Research Council for this work.

## REFERENCES

Alagendran, K., Hitch, D., Wadley, C. & Stagnitti, K. (2019). Cortisol responsivity to social play in children with autism: A systematic review. *Journal of Occupational Therapy, Schools, & Early Intervention*, 1-17.

Andersen, S., Kielhofner, G. & Lai, J. S. (2005). An examination of the measurement properties of the pediatric volitional questionnaire. *Physical & Occupational Therapy in Pediatrics*, *25*(1-2), 39-57.

Askins, L., Diasio, B., Szewerniak, D. & Cahill, S. M. (2013). Children with Developmental Disabilities and their Motivation to Play. *The Open Journal of Occupational Therapy*, *1*(4), 4.

Atieno, O. P. (2009). An analysis of the strengths and limitation of qualitative and quantitative research paradigms. *Problems of Education in the 21st Century*, *13*(1), 13-38.

Benitti, F. B. V. (2012). Exploring the educational potential of robotics in schools: A systematic review. *Computers & Education*, *58*(3), 978-988.

Boyd, L. E., Ringland, K. E., Haimson, O. L., Fernandez, H., Bistarkey, M. & Hayes, G. R. (2015). Evaluating a collaborative iPad game's impact on social relationships for children with autism spectrum disorder. *ACM Transactions on Accessible Computing (TACCESS)*, *7*(1), 3.

Bradt, J., Burns, D. S. & Creswell, J. W. (2013). Mixed methods research in music therapy research. *Journal of music therapy*, *50*(2), 123-148.

Cheng, C. C., Huang, P. L. & Huang, K. H. (2013). Cooperative learning in Lego robotics projects: Exploring the impacts of group formation on interaction and achievement. *Journal of Networks*, *8*(7), 1529.

Cohen, J. (1960). A coefficient of agreement for nominal scales. *Educational and psychological measurement*, *20*(1), 37-46.

Corrado, C. J. (1989). A nonparametric test for abnormal security-price performance in event studies. *Journal of financial economics*, *23*(2), 385-395.

Couch, K. J., Deitz, J. C. & Kanny, E. M. (1998). The role of play in pediatric occupational therapy. *American Journal of Occupational Therapy*, *52*(2), 111-117.

Creswell, J. W., Plano Clark, V. L., Gutmann, M. L. & Hanson, W. E. (2003). Advanced mixed methods research designs. *Handbook of Mixed Methods in Social and Behavioral Research*, *209*, 240.

Creswell, J. W., Shope, R., Plano Clark, V. L. & Green, D. O. (2006). How interpretive qualitative research extends mixed methods research. *Research in the Schools*, *13*(1), 1-11.

Elo, S. & Kyngäs, H. (2008). The qualitative content analysis process. *Journal of advanced nursing*, *62*(1), 107-115.

Fagerland, M. W. (2012). t-tests, non-parametric tests, and large studies—a paradox of statistical practice?. *BMC Medical Research Methodology*, *12*(1), 78.

Fertel-Daly, D., Bedell, G. & Hinojosa, J. (2001). Effects of a weighted vest on attention to task and self-stimulatory behaviors in preschoolers with pervasive developmental disorders. *American Journal of Occupational Therapy*, *55*(6), 629-640.

Fischer, H. E. & Neumann, K. (2012). Video analysis as a tool for understanding science instruction. In *Science Education Research and Practice in Europe*, (pp. 115-139): Springer.

Godin, J., Freeman, A. & Rigby, P. (2017). Interventions to promote the playful engagement in social interaction of preschool-aged children with autism spectrum disorder (ASD): a scoping study. *Early Child Development and Care*, 1-16.

Graneheim, U. H. & Lundman, B. (2004). Qualitative content analysis in nursing research: concepts, procedures and measures to achieve trustworthiness. *Nurse Education Today*, *24*(2), 105-112.

Groeneveld, R. A. & Meeden, G. (1984). Measuring skewness and kurtosis. *Journal of the Royal Statistical Society: Series D (The Statistician)*, *33*(4), 391-399.

Harper, C. B., Symon, J. B. & Frea, W. D. (2008). Recess is time-in: Using peers to improve social skills of children with autism. *Journal of autism and developmental disorders*, *38*(5), 815-826.

Harris, K. & Reid, D. (2005). The influence of virtual reality play on children's motivation. *Canadian Journal of Occupational Therapy*, *72*(1), 21-29.

Harrop, C., Green, J., Hudry, K. & Consortium, P. (2017). Play complexity and toy engagement in preschoolers with autism spectrum disorder: Do girls and boys differ? *Autism*, *21*(1), 37-50.

Hsieh, H. F. & Shannon, S. E. (2005). Three approaches to qualitative content analysis. *Qualitative Health Research*, *15*(9), 1277-1288.

Hunt, M. R. (2009). Strengths and Challenges in the Use of Interpretive Description: Reflections Arising From a Study of the Moral Experience of Health Professionals in Humanitarian Work. *Qualitative Health Research*, *19*(9), 1284-1292.

Huijnen, C. A., Lexis, M. A., Jansens, R. & de Witte, L. P. (2016). Mapping robots to therapy and educational objectives for children with autism spectrum disorder. *Journal of Autism and Developmental Disorders*, *46*(6), 2100-2114.

Hunt, M. R. (2009). Strengths and Challenges in the Use of Interpretive Description: Reflections Arising From a Study of the Moral Experience of Health Professionals in Humanitarian Work. *Qualitative Health Research*, *19*(9), 1284-1292.

Kolne, K. & Lindsay, S. (2019). Exploring Gender Differences in Teacher–Student Interactions during an Adapted Robotics Program for Children with Disabilities. *Social Sciences*, *8*(10), 285.

Krefting, L. (1991). Rigor in qualitative research: The assessment of trustworthiness. *American Journal of Occupational Therapy*, *45*(3), 214-222.

Lamptey, D. L., Cagliostro, E., Srikanthan, D., Hong, S., Dief, S. & Lindsay, S. (2019). Assessing the Impact of an Adapted Robotics Programme on Interest in Science, Technology, Engineering and Mathematics (STEM) among Children with Disabilities. *International Journal of Disability, Development and Education*, 1-16.

Law, M., King, G., King, S., Kertoy, M., Hurley, P., Rosenbaum, P., Young, N. & Hanna, S. (2006). Patterns of participation in recreational and leisure activities among children with complex physical disabilities. *Developmental medicine and child neurology*, *48*(5), 337-342.

LeGoff, D. B. (2004). Use of LEGO© as a therapeutic medium for improving social competence. *Journal of Autism and Developmental Disorders*, *34*(5), 557-571.

LeGoff, D. B. & Sherman, M. (2006). Long-term outcome of social skills intervention based on interactive LEGO© play. *Autism*, *10*(4), 317-329.

Libby, M. E., Weiss, J. S., Bancroft, S. & Ahearn, W. H. (2008). A comparison of most-to-least and least-to-most prompting on the acquisition of solitary play skills. *Behavior Analysis in Practice*, *1*(1), 37-43.

Lindsay, S. & Hounsell, K. G. (2017). Adapting a robotics program to enhance participation and interest in STEM among children with disabilities: a pilot study. *Disability and Rehabilitation: Assistive Technology*, *12*(7), 694-704.

Lindsay, S., Hounsell, K. & Cassiani, C. (2017). A scoping review of the role of LEGO. *Disabil Health Journal*, *10*(2), 173-182.

Lindsay, S. & Lam, A. (2017). Exploring types of play in an adapted robotics program for children with disabilities. *Disability and Rehabilitation: Assistive Technology*, 1-8.

Lindsay, S., McPherson, A. & Maxwell, J. (2017). Perspectives of school-work transitions among youth with spina bifida, their parents and health care providers. *Disability and Rehabilitation*, *39*(7), 641-652.

Lindsay, S., Ramptertab, L. & Curran, C. (2019). Therapy through play: Advancing the role of robotics in pediatric Rehabilitation. In *Everyday Technologies in HealthCare*, C. Hayre.

Liu, L., Pan, A., Chung, L., Gau, S., Kramer, J. & Lai, J. (2013). Reliability and validity of the Paediatric Volitional Questionnaire–Chinese version. *Journal of Rehabilitation Medicine*, *45*(1), 99-104.

Mayring, P. (2004). Qualitative content analysis. *A Companion to Qualitative Research*, *1*, 159-176.

McHugh, M. L. (2012). Interrater reliability: the kappa statistic. *Biochemia Medica*, *22*(3), 276-282.

Miller, S. & Reid, D. (2003). Doing play: competency, control, and expression. *Cyber Psychology & Behavior*, *6*(6), 623-632.

Noble, H. & Smith, J. (2015). Issues of validity and reliability in qualitative research. *Evidence-Based Nursing*, *18*(2), 34-35.

Peplak, J., Song, J. H., Colasante, T. & Malti, T. (2017). Only you can play with me! Children's inclusive decision making, reasoning, and emotions based on peers' gender and behavior problems. *Journal of Experimental Child Psychology*, *162*, 134-148.

Pizzamiglio, S., Naeem, U., Réhman, S., Saeed Sharif, M., Abdalla, H. & Turner, D. L. (2017). A Mutlimodal Approach to Measure the Distraction Levels of Pedestrians using Mobile Sensing. *Procedia Computer Science*, *113*, 89-96.

Pollock, N., Stewart, D., Law, M., Sahagian-Whalen, S., Harvey, S. & Toal, C. (1997). The meaning of play for young people with physical disabilities. *Canadian Journal of Occupational Therapy*, *64*(1), 25-31.

Rey, D. & Neuhäuser, M. (2011). Wilcoxon-Signed-Rank Test. In *International Encyclopedia of Statistical Science*. https://doi.org/10.1007/978-3-642-04898-2_616.

Salter, K., Beamish, W. & Davies, M. (2016). The effects of child-centered play therapy (CCPT) on the social and emotional growth of young Australian children with autism. *International Journal of Play Therapy*, *25*(2), 78.

Spiker, M. A., Lin, C. E., Van Dyke, M. & Wood, J. J. (2012). Restricted interests and anxiety in children with autism. *Autism*, *16*(3), 306-320.

Stephenson, J. & Carter, M. (2009). The use of weighted vests with children with autism spectrum disorders and other disabilities. *Journal of autism and developmental disorders*, *39*(1), 105.

Therrien, W. J., Wickstrom, K. & Jones, K. (2006). Effect of a combined repeated reading and question generation intervention on reading achievement. *Learning Disabilities Research & Practice*, *21*(2), 89-97.

Vaismoradi, M., Jones, J., Turunen, H. & Snelgrove, S. (2016). Theme development in qualitative content analysis and thematic analysis. *Journal of Nursing Education and Practice*, *6*(5), 100-110.

In: Understanding Children with Autism … ISBN: 978-1-53617-647-6
Editor: Anne Bourque 

*Chapter 5*

# ALTERED NEUROTRANSMITTER METABOLISM IN AUTISM SPECTRUM CONDITION

***Silvia Niñerola[1], Jordi Flores-Cervelló[1], Laura Campos-Berga[2], Isabel Torres-Cuevas[1], Máximo Vento[1,3] and Ana García-Blanco[3,4,*]***

[1]Neonatal Research Group, Health Research Institute La Fe, Valencia, Spain

[2]Division of Psychology, Hospital Universitari i Politècnic La Fe, Valencia, Spain

[3]Division of Neonatology, Hospital Universitari i Politècnic La Fe, Valencia, Spain

[4]Department of Personality, Evaluation and Psychological Treatment, University of Valencia, Valencia, Spain

[*] Corresponding Author's E-mail: ana.garcia-blanco@uv.es.

## Abstract

Autism spectrum condition (ASC) has been widely studied in literature, but many questions still need to be answered regarding how neurotransmitters are involved and how they are related to ASC psychopathology. A review was carried out in order to describe the main neurotransmitters in ASC patients. Among the studied neurotransmitters, increased serotonin and glutamate as well as decreased levels of gamma-aminobutyric acid N-Acetylaspartate and oxytocin appeared to have the most empirical evidence in ASC. Additional neurotransmitters as norepinephrine, acetylcholine, cortisol, and endogenous opioids have also been associated with ASC but there is still little support for the underlying mechanisms. Measurement of these neurotransmitters was usually obtained from different types of biological samples such as plasma, urine, or cerebrospinal fluid. Moreover, recent neuro-imaging techniques are also being used, providing a more precise and informative measure of neurotransmitter system functioning in ASC. Thus, several studies have described neurotransmitters' alterations in ASC patients. Overall, amino acid neurotransmitters, especially increased levels of serotonin, have shown more evidence for playing a role in ASC etiopathogenesis. Therefore, further neurotransmitter research is needed in order to elucidate the underlying mechanisms of ASC neuropathology, supporting a more comprehensive and theory-based approach of this disorder. Finally, measurement of these neurotransmitters and studies to search for new biomarkers may become a potential target for helping clinicians with early ASC diagnosis and treatment.

## 1. Introduction

Autism spectrum condition (ASC) is a neurodevelopmental disorder which is characterized by severe and sustained impairment in social interactions, abnormalities in verbal and non-verbal communication, restrictive or repetitive interests, and stereotyped behaviours and movements (American Psychiatric Association, 2013). The prevalence of ASC is 11,3 per 1000, with a male-to-female ratio of 3–4:1, over the last decade (U.S. Department of Health and Human Services, 2012). Being diagnosed at early stages of development could facilitate early interventions and therapies, benefiting both patients and their families (Sacrey, Bennett and

Zwaigenbaum, 2015; Zwaigenbaum et al., 2016). However, some subtle behavioural abnormalities are often overlooked in ASC infants and are not evident until approximately 12–18 months of age (Walsh et al., 2011; Wan et al., 2013). Regarding pathophysiological causes of ASC, genetic predisposition and environmental contributors have been implicated, with evidence that ASC is associated with abnormal brain development (Shimmura et al., 2011; Drenthen et al., 2016). But the neural mechanisms that could explain the aetiology of ASC are not yet completely understood (Barendse et al., 2013; Baruth et al., 2013). Since neurotransmitters play a major role in the central and peripheral nervous system development, these neuroactive amino acids are thought to be implicated in the pathogenesis and possible treatment of ASC. Thus, identifying and characterizing changes in their concentrations in body fluids is also important in case they may be relevant to the early diagnosis and intervention in ASC patients. This chapter reviews the literature on such measurements of the main neurotransmitters associated with ASC.

## 2. Neurotransmitters

### 2.1. Glutamatergic System

#### *2.1.1. Glutamate*

##### 2.1.1.1. Function

Glutamate is considered the major excitatory neurotransmitter and is highly concentrated throughout the central nervous system (CNS) (Shimmura et al., 2011). It plays an important role in brain development, affecting neuronal migration and plasticity, neuronal differentiation, survival, and synaptogenesis (Coyle, Leski and Morrison, 2002; Shinohe et al., 2006; Lodge, 2009). Glutamate is also crucial for the maintenance of cognitive processes such as memory, learning, behaviour, or motor activity (Manent and Represa, 2007). However, excess glutamate acts as a potent neurotoxin leading neuronal cells to death with deleterious consequences (Shimmura et al., 2011).

In recent years, there has been a growing interest in the role glutamatergic neurotransmission may play in the pathophysiology of ASC (Zheng et al., 2016). In fact, several studies including animal research, genetic determination, and postmortem analysis have reported that abnormal glutamate levels might be associated with a wide variety of neurobiological and behavioural alterations associated with autism, possibly related to an imbalance between neuronal excitation and inhibition (Won et al., 2012; Cai et al., 2016; Zheng et al., 2016). Interestingly, one study suggested that plasma glutamate levels can serve as a diagnostic tool for the early ASC detection, especially for normal IQ (Intelligence Quotient) autism forms (Shimmura et al., 2011; Cai et al., 2016).

#### 2.1.1.2. Levels

Although glutamate is reported to not easily cross the blood-brain barrier (Sheldon and Robinson, 2008). However, studies have shown that glutamate levels in blood are positively correlated with cerebrospinal fluid (CSF) levels of glutamate in humans (Shimmura et al., 2011). Recently, Hassan et al., (2013) reported a highly significant positive correlation between blood glutamate levels and brain glutamate levels. Thus, peripheral glutamate level can be used to reflect the glutamate level in the brain (Shimmura et al., 2011). This indirect measure of glutamate activity through blood samples is much easier to perform offering the possibility to use glutamate blood concentrations as a possible biological marker for ASC (Zheng et al., 2016).

#### 2.1.1.3. Proposed Mechanisms

Recently, a hypothesis based on evidence of an excessive neuronal excitation mediated by glutamate in ASC individuals has been proposed (Shimmura et al., 2011). Regarding pathophysiology of ASC, several studies have reported that blood glutamate levels are significantly higher in ASC individuals compared with Typical Development (TD) ones (Hassan et al., 2013; Cai et al., 2016; Drenthen et al., 2016; Zheng et al., 2016), which may reflect higher brain glutamate levels in ASC. In fact, previous studies using proton magnetic resonance spectroscopy (MRS) reported increased glutamate concentration in individuals with ASC (Brown et al., 2013; Joshi et al., 2013). For instance, Fatemi et al., (2002) registered reduced levels of GAD 65 kDa and GAD 67 kDa proteins, both involved in converting glutamate to Gamma-Aminobutyric Acid (GABA) and then resulting in increased levels of glutamate in the brain substrate. In addition, Page et al., (2006) has demonstrated that ASC individuals have significantly higher concentrations of glutamate in some brain regions (amygdala-hippocampal regions but not in parietal region) than TD controls. Shimmura et al., (2011) and Moreno-Fuenmayor et al. (1996) observed the same tendency of elevated plasma glutamate in ASC infants. Moreover, this elevation appears to be sustained over a long period of time, i.e., into adulthood (Shinohe et al., 2006). In fact, Shinohe et al., (2006) reported that high levels of glutamate are weakly associated with severity of ASC in terms of social interactions. Nevertheless, other studies have indicated no significant difference in glutamate levels between ASC individuals and controls (Zheng et al., 2016). This discrepancy may be due to methodological differences (e.g., time of sample collection, serum vs plasma, age of subjects) although the exactly reasons are currently unknown (Shinohe et al., 2006).

Although the causal mechanism of increased glutamate in ASC is not entirely recognized, several mechanisms have been considered. Firstly, elevated glutamate levels in the brain are related with metabolism dysregulation and increased gliosis in ASC patient's brains (Zheng et al., 2016). The increase of astroglial cells could be producing glutamate from glutamine via glutaminase enzyme, it seems reasonable to assume that an increase in number of glial cells may contribute to increase glutamate brain availability (Fatemi, 2008), which may alter enzymatic regulation disturbing the glutamatergic system/glutamate metabolism (Zheng et al., 2016). Secondly, levels of glutamic acid decarboxylase 65 and 67 kDa proteins are reduced in brains of ASC individuals (Fatemi et al., 2002). Since this enzyme is involved in converting glutamate to GABA, any reduction in its number or activity leads to increases in substrate compound glutamate in the brain. Owing to glutamate excitatory effects in brain, inducing activation by binding post-synaptic receptors, higher levels of glutamate may induce over-activity in the occipital region (Drenthen et al., 2016). Then, it has been speculated that higher levels of glutamate in ASC can be responsible for excitotoxicity, the process of damaging neurons due to the over-activity (Drenthen et al., 2016).

For the above-mentioned reasons, elevated plasma glutamate levels in ASC patients compared to TD controls support the hypothesis that hyperglutamatergic neurotransmission in the brain may contribute to ASC pathophysiology. Thus, blood glutamate levels may be considered as a potential biomarker in ASC diagnosis, although more comprehensive studies with large samples are needed to provide more conclusive results. Moreover, the effects of medications on peripheral glutamate levels and the correlation between the clinical symptoms in ASC and peripheral glutamate levels still need further investigation.

### *2.1.2. Glutamine*

#### 2.1.2.1. Function

Glutamine is the most abundant amino acid in plasma and it is a critical mitochondrial metabolic fuel for brain neurons and astrocytes (Good, 2011; Stelmashook et al., 2011). It exhibits extremely rapid cellular turnover rates and serves as an essential metabolic precursor in nucleotide, glucose and amino sugar biosynthesis, glutathione homeostasis, protein synthesis, and a source of oxidative energy (Tapiero et al., 2002). Glutamine, as a neurotransmitter, is involved in the glutamate-glutamine cycle, an important constituent of the glutamatergic neurotransmission system, in which glutamine is hydrolysed to glutamate in neurons, taken up into astrocytes, where is converted back into glutamine, and then returned to neurons to be stored and reused (Hesse and Mezger, 1978; Bak, Schousboe and Waagepetersen, 2006; Shimmura et al., 2013; Cochran et al., 2015; Zheng et al., 2017). Thus, glutamine exists as an intracellular buffer to prevent the excess of glutamate that does not participate in neurotransmission (Cochran et al., 2015). Thus, some studies suggest glutamine concentration could be a more sensitive measure of synaptic glutamatergic neurotransmission than glutamate itself (Pereira et al., 2008; Öngür et al., 2009; Cochran et al., 2015).

A meta-analysis of functional neuroimaging studies revealed that subjects with ASC showed greater probability of anterior cingulate cortex (ACC) hypoactivation compared with that of controls (Di Martino et al., 2008), which may be attributable to abnormalities in glutamatergic neurotransmission (Tekin and Cummings, 2002). In addition, several studies have demonstrated certain dysregulation in glutamate-glutamine metabolic cycle in ASC individuals, leading to impaired glutamate and glutamine levels in brain (Fatemi et al., 2002; Shimmura et al., 2013; Edmonson, Ziats and Rennert, 2014).

#### 2.1.2.2. Levels

Concerning glutamine concentrations, most published literature found decreased plasma glutamine concentration plasma (Moreno-Fuenmayor H, Borjas L, Arrieta A, Valera V, 1996; Aldred et al., 2003; Good, 2011; Shimmura et al., 2011; Tirouvanziam, Rabindra Obukhanych, Tetyana V. Laval et al., 2012; El-Ansary, 2016; Zheng et al., 2017) in ASC children compared with TD children (Ghanizadeh, 2013; Al-Otaish et al., 2018). In fact, detection of low plasma glutamine levels has been suggested as a screening test for ASC, especially useful in children with normal IQ (Shimmura et al., 2011; Ghanizadeh, 2013). Aldred et al., (2003) also found reduced levels of glutamine together with elevated levels of glutamate in plasma of ASC individuals. However, authors using other types of samples reported distinct results, with no significant differences between ASC and controls serum samples (Shinohe et al., 2006), or contradictory data with either increased (Noto et al., 2014) or decreased (Evans et al., 2008) glutamine levels in urine samples of ASC individuals.

Frequently, glutamate and glutamine are reported together as Glx due to difficulties in separating out the resonances. Majority proton magnetic resonance spectroscopy (1H-MRS) studies have found elevated levels of Glx although it depends on the brain region and individual's age (Cochran et al., 2015). In children and adolescents with ASC, Glx has been reported to be decreased in frontal and occipital grey matter and cerebellum (DeVito et al.,

2007), but increased in ACC (Bejjani et al., 2012). Additionally, in adults with ASC, Glx has been reported to be increased in amygdala/hippocampal region (Page et al., 2006) and auditory cortex (Brown et al., 2013) and decreased in the right ACC (Bernardi et al., 2011) and basal ganglia (Horder et al., 2013). However, another 1H-MRS study revealed no such difference in Glx in the ACC of ASC children (Shimmura et al., 2013). These inconsistent results might be attributable to differences in age range and/or the equipment resolution used (Shimmura et al., 2013).

Since glutamate and glutamine play a role in intermediary metabolism, other researchers suggest that their measurements either alone or together are not a particularly useful index of glutamatergic synaptic measure (Hall et al., 2015; Al-Otaish et al., 2018). Given glutamate synthesis occurs in neurons and glutamine synthesis in astrocytes, the glutamine/glutamate (Gln/Glu) ratio has been proposed as a more accurate and useful measure for quantifying neuronal–astrocyte interactions and glutamatergic metabolites balance (Hall et al., 2015; Al-Otaish et al., 2018). In fact, 1H-MRS studies in mood disorders support the idea of Gln/Glu ratio as a more accurate and sensitive marker of glutamatergic neurotransmission (Yüksel and Öngür, 2010; Cochran et al., 2015). Nevertheless, results are not consistent among literature in ASC. Some studies observed significantly higher Gln/Glu ratio in ASC patients compared to TD controls. In Al-Otaish et al.'s study, Glu/Gln ratio was 56.98% elevated in ASC children compared to TD control (Al-Otaish et al., 2018), which may reflect increased glutamate neurotransmission in ASC patients. Several MRS studies detected reduced Glu/Gln ratio in cortex and cerebellum of ASC boys (DeVito et al., 2007; Good, 2011) and also in right ACC of high-functioning ASC adults (Bernardi et al., 2011). Other studies like Page et al., (2006), found that Glu/Gln ratio was elevated in the amygdala-hippocampal region of ASC adults, but not altered in the parietal region (Page et al., 2006; Good, 2011). Shimmura et al. (2013) also described a lower Glu/Gln ratio in ASC samples compared with controls, although differences did not reach statistical significance (Good, 2011; Shimmura et al., 2013).

#### 2.1.2.3. Proposed Mechanisms

Concerning the role of glutamine neurotransmission on the pathophysiology of ASC, is important to consider the glutamate-glutamine cycle as a multicellular enzymatic process critical for maintaining synaptic function. Thus, an imbalance in any step of the cycle or in its metabolites free concentrations, could imply negative consequences in brain functions which contribute to developing several CNS disorders (Ortinski et al., 2010; Shimmura et al., 2011). In fact, there is evidence suggesting a link between glutamate-glutamine metabolism dysregulation and increased levels of gliosis in brains of ASC individuals. Moreover, Ortinski et al., (2010). found that activated astrocytes downregulate the expression of glutamine synthetase, the enzyme that converts glutamate into glutamine, which leads to reduced glutamine coupled with elevated glutamate (Ortinski et al., 2010). Another enzyme implicated in this cycle is glutaminase, which converts glutamine into glutamate and has been shown to be upregulated in activated microglia (Shimmura et al., 2011). Thus, it is suggested that gliosis process may be related to the aetiology of autism, as mediated by activated astrocytes and/or activated microglia, which may disturb the regulation of certain types of enzymes and thereby alter the glutamate-glutamine metabolism (Shimmura et al., 2011).

To sum up, glutamine is a neurotransmitter which plays a crucial role in maintaining brain glutamatergic system due to its function of preventing excessive levels of glutamate, by a glutamate-glutamine cycle in cerebral neurons and astrocytes. It seems that alterations in glutamine levels, particularly reduced concentrations, produce an imbalance in this system which appears to affect some brain functions impaired in ASC. Some research suggests that glutamine measure is more sensitive and reflects synaptic glutamatergic neurotransmission better that glutamate. But other authors propose calculating Glu/Gln ratio or measuring it together with glutamate, as Glx. However, there is still inconclusive results and is needed to provide further evidence about how impaired glutamine levels affect brain functioning of ASC individuals.

## 2.2. GABA

### *2.2.1. Function*

GABA is regarded as the main inhibitory neurotransmitter in adult human and mammalian brain (Coghlan et al., 2012) as 25–40% of all axon terminals contain GABA (Dhossche et al., 2002). Thus, it is responsible for most inhibitory communication in the brain (Lam, Aman and Arnold, 2006). Whereas in the adult brain GABA acts as an inhibitory neurotransmitter, it also plays an important role as an excitatory neurotransmitter in several neurodevelopmental processes since early stages (Van Kooten, Hof and Engeland, 2005; Sibilla and Ballerini, 2009; El-Ansary and Al-Ayadhi, 2014; Al-Otaish et al., 2018)GABA promotes events such as neuronal migration, proliferation and differentiation, synapse maturation and cell death (Owens and Kriegstein, 2002; Van Kooten, Hof and Engeland, 2005; Sibilla and Ballerini, 2009; Al-Otaish et al., 2018). GABA is an amino acid transmitter synthesised from the excitatory neurotransmitter glutamate via glutamate decarboxylase (GAD) enzymes, and released by inhibitory interneurons (Coghlan et al., 2012). Inhibitory interneurons have small dimensions and projection areas (Coghlan et al., 2012), and they are present in a relatively low number (10–15% of neuronal population). In spite of that, these neurons synchronize a large number of principal cells giving rise to coherent oscillations, which supports different behavioural states and high cognitive tasks (Klausberger and Somogyi, 2008; Cellot and Cherubini, 2014). Altogether, these observations point to GABA as one of the major players in the early assembly and formation of neuronal circuits in the developing brain (Cellot and Cherubini, 2014). Therefore, a dysfunction of GABAergic signalling at early development may lead to a severe excitatory/inhibitory (E/I) imbalance in neuronal circuits (Pizzarelli and Cherubini, 2011; El-Ansary and Al-Ayadhi, 2014) affecting neural signalling and transmission, and thus behavioural and socio-cognitive functions (Cellot and Cherubini, 2014; Ford and Crewther, 2016; Canitano and Pallagrosi, 2017; Ford, Abu-Akel and Crewther, 2019).

Several studies defend an important role of GABA in ASC aetiology or pathophysiology suggesting a clear E/I imbalance in selective neuronal circuits (Cellot and Cherubini, 2014; Ford, Abu-Akel and Crewther, 2019). This imbalanced ratio may be due to increased glutamate activity, decreased GABA release, or reduced GABA receptors in different brain structures (Rosenberg, Patterson and Angelaki, 2015; Al-Otaish et al., 2018). ASC symptomatology may be linked to the suppression of normal GABAergic inhibition, resulting in excessive stimulation of glutamate specialized neurons and loss of sensory gating (Hussman, 2001). In fact, data from animal models of ASC indicate that a dysfunction in GABAergic signalling may account for most of the ASC symptoms (Cellot and Cherubini, 2014). More direct evidence as genetic abnormalities observations, *in vitro* analysis of post-mortem brain tissues (reporting structural changes in both excitatory glutamatergic and inhibitory GABAergic circuits) and *In vivo* studies on patients affected mainly by idiopathic forms of ASCs, are in favour of a decreased or abnormal GABA inhibition in ASC (Hussman, 2001; Dhossche et al., 2002; Cellot and Cherubini, 2014; Canitano and Pallagrosi, 2017).

#### *2.2.2. Levels*

GABA levels have been less studied due to the specialized editing techniques needed to segregate the GABA content (Cochran et al., 2015). There are 1H-MRS brain studies published (DeVito et al., 2007; Harel-Gadassi et al., 2018); however, given the difficulties in distinguishing GABA from other similar molecules with MRS, only some studies have estimate concentrations of GABA in children with ASC using 1H-MRS (Coghlan et al., 2012; Cochran et al., 2015). These studies found decreased GABA levels in frontal lobe (Harada et al., 2011), as well as in auditory (Gaetz et al., 2014; Rojas et al., 2014), and motor (Gaetz et al., 2014) cortices. Regarding GABA concentrations in plasma, few and inconclusive results have been found between different works. Thus, some studies reported increased GABA in plasma of ASC individuals (Dhossche et al., 2002; El-Ansary, Bacha and Ayahdi, 2011). However, Borgatti, Piccinelli and Passoni (2001) reported no significant differences in plasmatic GABA levels between ASC children and TD controls, and even Rolf et al., (1993) observed decreased GABA levels in platelets. About postmortem studies providing evidence of altered GABAergic circuits in ASC individuals

(Canitano and Pallagrosi, 2017), Fatemi et al., (2002) measured brain levels of GAD enzyme, which is considered the rate-limiting step in the synthesis of GABA. They found that GAD was reduced in ASC patients by 48–61% in parietal and cerebellar areas when compared to controls. Other studies have reported reduced expression of GABAergic genes and reduced density of GABA-related proteins in postmortem brain samples from ASC individuals (Coghlan et al., 2012).

In view of the difficult measurement of GABA levels and its relation to glutamate metabolism (one derives from each other, and therefore alterations in one neurotransmitter can affect the other) (Al-Otaish et al., 2018), some studies measure glutamate/GABA ratio instead of GABA levels alone. This index was significantly higher in ASC patients compared to controls, thus suggesting a possible abnormality in glutamate/GABA regulation. It might lead to excitotoxicity which in turn may manifest behaviourally through social difficulties (El-Ansary and Al-Ayadhi, 2014). In fact, Ford, Nibbs and Crewther (2017) reported higher socio-cognitive difficulties associated with higher glutamate/GABA ratio in the right superior temporal lobe in ASC.

### *2.2.3. Proposed Mechanisms*

Despite elevated GABA in plasma of ASC patients, findings of reduced density of GABA receptors in the hippocampus (El-Ansary and Al-Ayadhi, 2014; El-Ansary, 2016) is supportive with the hypothesis of dysfunction in inhibitory GABAergic system, resulting in excessive stimulation of the glutamate system (Lam, Aman and Arnold, 2006) which in turn, influences neuronal growth and connectivity during early development (Ford, Abu-Akel and Crewther, 2019).

Several studies have suggested altered GABA function in ASC, although the pathophysiological origin of these alterations remains unclear (Puts et al., 2017). Some genetic studies have reported abnormalities in the proximal arm of chromosome 15 (15q11-13) in ASC individuals (Van Kooten, Hof and Engeland, 2005). This site contains genes coding for particular subunits of the GABAA receptor (Cook et al., 1998; Martin et al., 2000), which can be the reason of the difficulties in the assembly of GABAA receptor reported in some brain areas of ASC individuals (Dhossche et al., 2002). Other possible explanation proposed by Dhossche et al., (2002) is that elevated GABA plasma levels could reflect a compensatory increase in presynaptic GABA release in response to hyposensitivity of a subset of GABA receptors. This in turn could produce increased postsynaptic activation of other normal GABA receptor subtypes, resulting in complex alterations of GABAergic function throughout the brain, leading to neurologic and behavioural problems, including hyperactivity and epilepsy, frequent comorbidities in ASC (Dhossche et al., 2002; Van Kooten, Hof and Engeland, 2005).

In summary, although there is little research examining GABA system in living human brains, due to technical limitations, in recent years such studies have begun to provide preliminary evidence consistent with GABA abnormalities in ASC individuals compared to TD controls (Coghlan et al., 2012). New studies about the mechanism by which GABA can be implicated in the neuropathophysiology of ASC would allow the development of specific drugs for ASC treatment. In fact, several studies have shown that drugs acting on GABAergic synapses are able to correct behavioural deficits in animal models of ASC and ameliorate at least some of ASC symptoms (Cellot and Cherubini, 2014).

## 2.3. Oxytocin

### *2.3.1. Function*

Oxytocin is a neuropeptide produced in the CNS and in peripheric tissues. This neurotransmitter is directly implicated in such crucial functions like bonding, processing emotions and stablishing social relations with other individuals (Carter, 2017). It also plays a relevant role in metabolism maintenance as well as in general energy balance through the body (Zhang et al., 2018).

### *2.3.2. Levels*

Measuring oxytocin blood levels has been the method of choice in many studies to determine its concentration in the CNS (Modahl et al., 1998), whose measurement improved other kinds of more invasive practices (like lumbar puncture). In addition, it has been shown that oxytocin levels in plasma and in CSF are strongly positively correlated (Carson et al., 2014), therefore an indirect assessment of oxytocin in the CNS can be performed.

Given its functions in the CNS, oxytocin has been hypothesised to play an important role in ASC pathophysiology. Many studies have successfully linked ASC with altered genes involved in oxytocin metabolism and oxytocin receptors in neurons as well as with altered oxytocin blood levels (Tan et al., 2019; Voinsky et al., 2019). Some studies have also linked ASC clinical severity in early age patients to circulating oxytocin blood levels (Kobylinska et al., 2019). Many studies have reported lower oxytocin blood levels in children suffering from ASC compared with age-matched TD groups (Modahl et al., 1998; Kobylinska et al., 2019), which reflects lower oxytocin levels acting in the CNS in ASC patients. However, some other studies show no significant differences when comparing blood oxytocin levels between ASC patients and the control group (Rutigliano et al., 2016). Moreover, other studies indicated that oxytocin blood levels were associated with the ASC symptoms severity (Husarova et al., 2016). Methodological differences (e.g., sample collection methods, number of patients) may be the reason for these discrepancies.

### *2.3.3. Proposed Mechanisms*

Different mechanisms by which this oxytocin deficit could affect patients suffering ASC have been described. Oxytocin is considered a modulator of other neurotransmitters like GABA, and its release may modulate the flux of information processed in the hippocampal region (Lopatina et al., 2018), which is responsible for emotional processing and motivation among other functions (Rajmohan and Mohandas, 2019). Low oxytocin levels correlate with imbalances of the E/I pathways regulated by other neurotransmitters given its neuromodulator role over other neuropeptides. In addition, when exogenous oxytocin was administrated intranasally to ASC patients –with lower oxytocin levels, researchers observed both acute and long-term favourable results regarding empathy and emotions perception, suggesting that low oxytocin levels are involved in those mental processes (Guastella et al., 2010; Anagnostou et al., 2012).

In conclusion, findings on lower oxytocin plasma levels in ASC patients may explain its involvement in ASC pathophysiology. Moreover, differences or changes in neurotransmitter levels in patients with a diagnosed ASC seems to be associated with the severity of the disorder and then may be useful for classification. Although further studies on the field are needed to obtain more precise and conclusive results, oxytocin can be considered a good potential biomarker given its easy measurement and its involved relation with ASC.

## 2.4. Serotonin

### *2.4.1. Function*

Serotonin, also known as 5-hydroxytryptamine (5-HT), is a neurotransmitter produced in the CNS and other tissues like the digestive system and blood (Lv and Liu, 2017). Serotonin regulates cognition, learning and memory, feelings like wellbeing and happiness as well as some social behaviours when acting in the CNS (Lv and Liu, 2017). In peripheral tissues, serotonin has been proven to act as a regulator for the survival of red blood cells in mice (Amireault et al., 2011) and to bind platelets which could enhance platelet activity (Dale et al., 2002). Serotonin has also been hypothesised to play a role in neurogenesis and neuroprotection in the hippocampus (Cowen, 2007).

### *2.4.2. Levels*

Due to its various functions in CNS, serotonin has been hypothesised to play a major role in ASC lately. Several studies including post-mortem analysis, animal research, and genetic tests indicate an existing link between serotonin and the ASC pathophysiology (Hranilovic et al., 2007; Kolevzon et al., 2010). Thus, induced brain hyperserotonaemia (elevated serotonin) in mice may be responsible for some ASC behaviours (Tanaka et al., 2018). In humans, specifically blood serotonin associated with platelets and urinary serotonin levels have been related to many symptoms and behaviours exhibited by ASC patients (Hranilovic et al., 2007)

Though serotonin is well known as neurotransmitter, most of serotonin body's supply is produced in peripheral tissues (Mück-Seler and Pivac, 2011). Studies carried out in mice showed no correlation between blood and brain serotonin (Pietraszek et al., 1992). However, ASC even though blood and brain serotonin levels did not match in previous animal studies, measuring blood serotonin levels could still be considered an interesting approach for ASC diagnosis and research. It has been described that brain serotonin levels are lowered in patients with ASC compared with healthy controls (Mcbride et al., 1988), and that high blood serotonin does not mean equivalent levels of serotonin in the brain but the opposite (Mcbride et al., 1988), as explained below.

Regarding blood samples, high platelet-associated serotonin levels have been linked to ASC (Gabriele, Sacco and Persico, 2014). It is discussed whether platelet serotonin is related to the ASC severity. In studies with adults, platelet serotonin was found significantly higher for the ASC group in comparison with the control one, supporting the hypothesis that blood hyperserotonaemia may be related to ASC (Hranilovic et al., 2007). Even though, serotonin levels were not found to correlate with severity of the ASC symptoms in adults (Hranilovic et al., 2007). Other studies performed on ASC children found that blood serotonin concentration was correlated with the ASC severity (Abdulamir, Abdul-Rasheed and Abdulghani, 2018). There is a trend indicating a positive correlation between blood serotonin-platelet associated levels and ASC clinic, nevertheless, results are still unclear.

### *2.4.3. Proposed Mechanisms*

Although the exact causal mechanisms ASC are not completely known, there are many biochemical interactions that could explain the role of serotonin in ASC pathophysiology. Increased serotonin is a consistent biomarker in ASC patients being presented in 25% of the cases approximately (Gabriele, Sacco and Persico, 2014). This hyperserotonaemia seems to be induced by an excess serotonin intake by platelets, leaving free circulating serotonin unaffected (Muller and Anacker, 2015). In addition, high serotonin levels could be explained by a) increased production in peripheral tissues, b) poor metabolic breakdown, or c) serotonin transporter malfunction due to genetic polymorphisms. Regarding serotonin transporters, some studies have been found them elevated in ASC patients (Alabdali, Al-Ayadhi and El-Ansary, 2014), which could be directly involved with a lower binding capacity of the transporter and its ligand. Then this would lead to low serotonin levels in brain despite high serotonin blood concentrations (deficit in transportation). Many studies support that brain serotonin levels are lowered in ASC patients compared with TD controls (Mcbride et al., 1988), and that high blood serotonin does not mean equivalent levels of serotonin in the brain but the opposite (Mcbride et al., 1988). Low brain serotonin levels affect social behaviours and emotional processing, symptoms presented by patients with ASC, with demonstrated defects in early neurogenesis (Patrick and Ames, 2014).

In conclusion, higher platelet-associated serotonin levels in blood could be considered an ASC biomarker given the tendency observed in autism cases. New studies are needed in order to get a better understanding of potential explicative factors of serotonin peripheral/central metabolism and its impact on ASC-like behaviours. Despite limited data, serotoninergic neurotransmission seems to be a promising target biomarker for early ASC diagnose and for future therapies and specific treatments of the disorder.

## 2.5. N-Acetylaspartate

### *2.5.1. Function*

N-acetylaspartate (NAA) is a derivative of aspartic acid, which is mostly synthetized and found in the CNS. The NAA physiological role in the brain is not well defined but highly discussed. It has been linked with early postnatal neuronal myelinization, as a key precursor for energy obtention and as an indicator of brain injury when found concentration reduced (Davie et al., 1994; Moffett et al., 2007). It has also been associated with Canavan disease, a rare but fatal neurodegenerative disorder (Bartalini et al., 1992).

### *2.5.2. Levels*

NAA levels can be measured directly in the CNS without any fluid extraction but using MRS thanks to its prominent proton signal (Moffett et al., 2007). Using this technique, NAA concentration is detected in specific brain regions. Moreover, fluctuations in those NAA levels over time could as well be observed and studied using MRS. It is important to remark that NAA cannot cross the blood-brain barrier, so blood sampling results ineffective to measure NAA central levels (Bogner-Strauss, 2017).

NAA has been hypothesised to be involved in ASC and its pathophysiology too. Several studies including ASC patients have reported abnormal levels of NAA in certain brain regions like the frontal lobe (Kleinhans et al., 2007). Many post-mortem studies also reported abnormalities in neuron count in some brain regions like the frontal lobe and cerebellum (Palmen et al., 2004). Disturbed NAA levels can lead to neuronal dysfunction or even neuronal loss, which could ultimately lead to behavioural and cognitional impairment present in ASC patients.

In the latest years, MRS studies showed a decrease of NAA levels in brain regions of ASC patients. Some studies revealed that NAA is decreased in the left frontal lobe cortex in ASC patients of different ages (Kleinhans et al., 2007; Carvalho Pereira et al., 2018). Moreover, a semi-partial correlation was found between NAA levels and frontal lobe activation in ASC individuals (Kleinhans et al., 2007). However, other studies showed no differences in NAA levels in the left frontal lobe between the ASC and the control groups (Hisaoka et al., 2001). These discrepancies could be explained by methodological differences and/or by ASC heterogeneity, since not all ASC patients present frontal lobe abnormalities when they are compared to control individuals (Kleinhans et al., 2007).

### *2.5.3. Proposed Mechanisms*

As explained before, NAA deficiency in some brain regions may imply lower neuron density or dysfunction of the existent neurons. Frontal lobe is responsible for incorporating cognitive and emotional processes, being crucial for normal emotional and intellectual development (Hoffmann, 2013). When NAA imbalance affects the frontal lobe (as observed in some ASC patients), those cognitive and behavioural functions could result impaired, leading to symptomatology expression observed in ASC patients (Ha et al., 2015). Other brain regions affected by a deficiency of NAA could further explain some other social and cognitive difficulties exhibited by ASC patients as well.

In conclusion, low NAA levels in some brain regions like the frontal lobe could explain some of ASC symptoms. Although not all ASC patients show NAA disturbances, NAA should still be taken into account as a potential biomarker for ASC diagnosis and characterisation. Further research is needed in order to define the role of NAA in ASC pathophysiology and perhaps design specific treatments and therapies in cases of NAA insufficiency.

## 2.6. Others

There are several studies that tried to establish consistent tendency patterns about levels of additional neurotransmitters. However, there is still inconsistent and contradictory results that did not allow to extract a clear conclusion about the paper and the levels tendency of them in ASC patients. Therefore, is still necessary more research on these neurotransmitters until they can be considered as good ASC biomarkers.

Among other potential ASC biomarkers, Taurine is a critical brain aminoacid that acts as an inhibitory transmitter and intracellular Ca2+ regulator (Good, 2011). It plays an important role in several essential biological processes and it has been shown to prevent oxidant-induced damage (Park and Cohen, 2017). Thus, is an osmoregulator and neuromodulator that suppresses vasopressin and has been reported to be augmented or decreased depending on the type of sample of autistic patients from it is measured (Zheng et al., 2017). In urine samples it has been found to be increased (Yap et al., 2010; Nadal-Desbarats et al., 2014), decreased

(Ming et al., 2012) or even depleted (Good, 2011) in ASC patients compared to healthy controls. In plasma samples there is also contradictory results, in fact, plasma levels have been reported to be increased (Moreno-Fuenmayor H, Borjas L, Arrieta A, Valera V, 1996; Shimmura et al., 2011; Kuwabara et al., 2013) or decreased (Geier et al., 2009; Kern et al., 2011; Tu, Chen and He, 2012). Nevertheless, there is a consistent opinion that taurine plays a protective role in patients with ASD (Good, 2011).

Cortisol, one of the most widely used physiological indicators of stress (Corbett et al., 2006), has been also studied as ASC biomarker and it has been evaluated to assess the theory that some of the related behavioural disturbances could be due to a chronic heightened level of activation and hyperarousal, which might result in elevated levels of this stress hormone (Lam, Aman and Arnold, 2006). Most of the published reports examining HPA responsiveness in ASC children have serious methodological weaknesses, which include a lack of appropriate controls, invasive sampling techniques, mixed diagnosis and very small samples, which leads to inconclusive and contradictory results when measuring basal levels. In fact, some studies found that baseline levels of cortisol functioning are not altered in ASC individuals compared to controls. Indeed, Bouvard et al. (1995) and Hill et al. (1977) have reported lower cortisol levels in plasma from ASC subjects compared to controls and aversely, Tordjman et al. (1997) found higher levels in individuals with severe ASC. In addition, Corbett et al. (2006) found that most children with ASC show more variation in daytime patterns of cortisol and significant elevations in salivary cortisol in response to a non-social stressor.

Glycine is, with GABA, the major inhibitory neurotransmitter in the CNS. Both, GABA and glycine depolarize membrane potentials, acting as excitatory neurotransmitters during early development (Zheng et al., 2017). Compared with healthy controls, glycine levels in ASC individuals have been reported to be unchanged in plasma (Tirouvanziam, Rabindra Obukhanych, Tetyana V. Laval et al., 2012) et al. 2011) and serum (Shinohe et al., 2006). Adversely, in urine samples glycine levels have been reported to be increased (Noto et al., 2014) but also decreased (Evans et al., 2008; Ming et al., 2012).

Other studied molecules are amino acids as tryptophan, which is the precursor of serotonin. In contrast to what have been reported for serotonin, tryptophan levels in plasma have been reported to be decreased in ASC (Tirouvanziam, Rabindra Obukhanych, Tetyana V. Laval et al., 2012; Tu, Chen and He, 2012; Naushad et al., 2013). Nevertheless, studies measuring tryptophan from urine samples reported increased tryptophan levels (Noto et al., 2014) but in other studies reported them to be decreased (Kałuzna-Czaplińska et al., 2014). Other amino acids (such as glycine, tryptophan or d-serine) could also be involved and it may be important to carry out comprehensive studies in which a number of these amino acids are investigated simultaneously in order to avoid considerable variation in terms of factors such as age, gender, number of subjects or psychoactive medication being taken (Zheng et al., 2017).

## Conclusion

The hypothesis of an impaired amino acid neurotransmission in ASC is supported by several research findings based on neuroanatomic and neurobiological analysis. Many studies reported higher glutamate and serotonin plasma levels in ASC patients compared with controls, whereas levels of glutamine, oxytocin, and NAA were frequently lower in ASC groups. Moreover, several ASC functional deficits are consistent with an E/I imbalance caused by either increased glutamatergic (excitatory neurotransmitter) signalling or reduced GABAergic (mainly inhibitory neurotransmitter) signalling. That biochemical imbalance has been proposed as one of the main pathopsychological causes of ASC. In addition, the limbic structures, the frontal cortex, and the cerebellum appear to be particularly relevant as well due to their important role in sensory input integration.

Measurement of these neurotransmitters was usually obtained from different types of biological samples; however, plasma samples seems to provide more consistent and solid results among published literature. Moreover, recent neuro-imaging techniques are also being used, providing a more precise and informative measure of neurotransmitter system functioning in ASC.

Nevertheless, the results reported in the literature are generally contradictory and inconclusive. This variation is probably due to methodological differences in sampling factors such as sex, age, sample size, IQ, type of biological sample, etc. Therefore, future studies should include simultaneous analyses of a large number of amino acids and standardization of the mentioned factors. Moreover, little is known yet about the underlying mechanisms that could explain ASC pathophysiology and symptomatology expression. Finally, more research on neurotransmitters is needed also relating its potential use as biomarkers, which could allow an early ASC diagnose and therapeutic intervention.

## REFERENCES

Abdulamir, H. A., Abdul-Rasheed, O. F. & Abdulghani, E. A. (2018). 'Serotonin and serotonin transporter levels in autistic children', *Saudi Medical Journal*, *39*(5), pp. 487–494. doi: 10.15537/smj.2018.5.21751.

Al-Otaish, H., et al. (2018). 'Relationship between absolute and relative ratios of glutamate, glutamine and GABA and severity of autism spectrum disorder', *Metabolic Brain Disease*. Metabolic Brain Disease, *33*(3), pp. 843–854. doi: 10.1007/s11011-018-0186-6.

Alabdali, A., Al-Ayadhi, L. & El-Ansary, A. (2014). 'Association of social and cognitive impairment and biomarkers in autism spectrum disorders', *Journal of Neuroinflammation*, *11*, pp. 1–14. doi: 10.1186/ 1742-2094-11-4.

Aldred, S., et al. (2003). 'Plasma amino acid levels in children with autism and their families', *Journal of Autism and Developmental Disorders*, *33*(1), pp. 93–97. doi: 10.1023/A:1022238706604.

American Psychiatric Association. (2013). 'American Psychiatric Association. Diagnostic and Statistical Manual of Mental Disorders. 5th ed', in *American Psychiatric Association*.

Amireault, P., et al. (2011). 'Ineffective erythropoiesis with reduced red blood cell survival in serotonin-deficient mice', *Proceedings of the National Academy of Sciences of the United States of America*, *108*(32), pp. 13141–13146. doi: 10.1073/pnas.

Anagnostou, E., et al. (2012). 'Intranasal oxytocin versus placebo in the treatment of adults with autism spectrum disorders: A randomized controlled trial', *Molecular Autism*, *3*(16), pp. 1–9. doi: 10.1186/2040-2392-3-16.

Bak, L. K., Schousboe, A. & Waagepetersen, H. S. (2006). 'The glutamate/GABA-glutamine cycle: Aspects of transport, neurotransmitter homeostasis and ammonia transfer', *Journal of Neurochemistry*, pp. 641–653. doi: 10.1111/j.1471-4159.2006.03913.x.

Barendse, E. M., et al. (2013). 'Working memory deficits in high-functioning adolescents with autism spectrum disorders: neuropsychological and neuroimaging correlates', *Journal of Neurodevelopmental Disorders*, *5*(14), pp. 1–11. doi: 10.1186/1866-1955-5-14.

Bartalini, G., et al. (1992). 'Biochemical diagnosis of Canavan disease', *Child's Nervous System*, *8*, pp. 468–470. doi: 10.1007/BF00274411.

Baruth, J. M., et al. (2013). 'Proton Magnetic Resonance Spectroscopy as a Probe into the Pathophysiology of Autism Spectrum Disorders (ASD): A Review', *Autism Research*, *6*(2), pp. 119–133. doi: 10.1002/ aur.1273.

Bejjani, A., et al. (2012). 'Elevated glutamatergic compounds in pregenual anterior cingulate in pediatric autism spectrum disorder demonstrated by1H MRS and 1H MRSI', *PLoS ONE*, *7*(7), p. e38786. doi: 10.1371/journal.pone.0038786.

Bernardi, S., et al. (2011). '*In vivo* 1 H-magnetic resonance spectroscopy study of the attentional networks in autism', *Brain Research*. Elsevier B.V., 1380, pp. 198–205. doi: 10.1016/j.brainres.2010.12.057.

Bogner-Strauss, J. G. (2017). 'N-acetylaspartate metabolism outside the brain: Lipogenesis, histone acetylation, and cancer', *Frontiers in Endocrinology*, *8*(240), pp. 1–5. doi: 10.3389/fendo.2017.00240.

Borgatti, R., et al. (2001). 'Pervasive Developmental Disorders and GABAergic System in Patients With Inverted Duplicated Chromosome 15', *Journal of Child Neurology*, *16*(12), pp. 911–914.

Bouvard, M. P., et al. (1995). 'Low-dose naltrexone effects on plasma chemistries and clinical symptoms in autism: a double-blind, placebo-controlled study', *Psychiatry Research*, *58*(3), pp. 191–201. doi: 10.1016/0165-1781(95)02601-R.

Brown, M. S., et al. (2013). 'Increased glutamate concentration in the auditory cortex of persons with autism and first-degree relatives: A 1H-MRS study', *Autism Research*, *6*(1), pp. 1–10. doi: 10.1002/aur.1260.

Cai, J., et al. (2016). 'Elevated plasma levels of glutamate in children with autism spectrum disorders', *NeuroReport*, *27*(4), pp. 272–276. doi: 10.1097/WNR.0000000000000532.

Canitano, R. & Pallagrosi, M. (2017). 'Autism spectrum Disorders and schizophrenia spectrum Disorders : excitation/inhibition imbalance and Developmental trajectories', *Frontiers in Psychiatry*, *8*(69), pp. 1–7. doi: 10.3389/fpsyt.2017.00069.

Carson, D. S., et al. (2014). 'Cerebrospinal fluid and plasma oxytocin concentrations are positively correlated and negatively predict anxiety in children', *Molecular Psychiatry*. Nature Publishing Group, *20*(9), pp. 1085–1090. doi: 10.1038/mp.2014.132.

Carter, C. S. (2017). 'The role of oxytocin and vasopressin in attachment', *Psychodynamic Psychiatry, 45*(4), pp. 499–518. doi: 10.1521/pdps.2017.45.4.499.

Carvalho Pereira, A., et al. (2018). 'Medial Frontal Lobe Neurochemistry in Autism Spectrum Disorder is Marked by Reduced N-Acetylaspartate and Unchanged Gamma-Aminobutyric Acid and Glutamate + Glutamine Levels', *Journal of Autism and Developmental Disorders*. Springer US, *48*(5), pp. 1467–1482. doi: 10.1007/s10803-017-3406-8.

Cellot, G. & Cherubini, E. (2014). 'GABAergic signaling as therapeutic target for autism spectrum disorders', *Frontiers in Pediatrics*, pp. 1–11. doi: 10.3389/fped.2014.00070.

Cochran, D. M., et al. (2015). 'Relationship among Glutamine, c-Aminobutyric Acid, and Social Cognition in Autism Spectrum

Disorders', *J Child Adolesc Psychopharmacol.*, *25*(4), pp. 314–322. doi: 10.1089/cap.2014.0112.

Coghlan, S., et al. (2012). 'GABA System Dysfunction in Autism and Related Disorders: From Synapse to Symptoms', *Neurosci Biobehav Rev*, *36*(9), pp. 2044–2055. doi: 10.1016/j.neubiorev.2012.07.005.

Cook, E. H., et al. (1998). 'Linkage-disequilibrium mapping of autistic disorder, with 15q11-13 markers', *American Journal of Human Genetics*, *62*(5), pp. 1077–1083. doi: 10.1086/301832.

Corbett, B. A., et al. (2006). 'Cortisol circadian rhythms and response to stress in children with autism', *Psychoneuroendocrinology*, *31*(1), pp. 59–68. doi: 10.1016/j.psyneuen.2005.05.011.

Cowen, D. S. (2007). 'Serotonin and neuronal growth factors - A convergence of signaling pathways', *Journal of Neurochemistry*, *101*(5), pp. 1161–1171. doi: 10.1111/j.1471-4159.2006.04420.x.

Coyle, J. T., Leski, M. L. & Morrison, J. H. (2002). 'The diverse roles of L-glutamic acid in brain signal transduction.', *Neuropsychopharmacology, The Fifth Generation of Progress*, pp. 71–90.

Dale, G. L., et al. (2002). 'Stimulated platelets use serotonin to enhance their retention of procoagulant proteins on the cell surface', *Nature*, pp. 175–179. doi: 10.1038/415175a.

Davie, C. A., et al. (1994). 'Serial proton magnetic resonance spectroscopy in acute multiple sclerosis lesions', *Brain*, *117*(1), pp. 49–58. doi: 10.1093/brain/117.1.49.

DeVito, T. J., et al. (2007). 'Evidence for Cortical Dysfunction in Autism: A Proton Magnetic Resonance Spectroscopic Imaging Study', *Biological Psychiatry*, *61*(4), pp. 465–473. doi: 10.1016/j.biopsych.2006.07.022.

Dhossche, D., et al. (2002). 'Elevated plasma gamma-aminobutyric acid (GABA) levels in autistic youngsters: Stimulus for a GABA hypothesis of autism', *Medical Science Monitor*, *8*(8), pp. 1–7.

Drenthen, G. S., et al. (2016) 'Altered neurotransmitter metabolism in adolescents with high- functioning autism Gerhard', *Psychiatry Res.*, *256*, pp. 44–49. doi: 10.1097/CCM.0b013e31823da96d.Hydrogen.

Edmonson, C., Ziats, M. N. & Rennert, O. M. (2014). 'Altered glial marker expression in autistic post-mortem prefrontal cortex and cerebellum', *Molecular Autism*, *5*(3), pp. 1–9. doi: 10.1186/2040-2392-5-3.

El-Ansary, A. (2016). 'Data of multiple regressions analysis between selected biomarkers related to glutamate excitotoxicity and oxidative stress in Saudi autistic patients', *Data in Brief*. Elsevier, 7, pp. 111–116. doi: 10.1016/j.dib.2016.02.025.

El-Ansary, A. & Al-Ayadhi, L. (2014). 'GABAergic/glutamatergic imbalance relative to excessive neuroinflammation in autism spectrum disorders', *Journal of Neuroinflammation*, *11*(189), pp. 1–9. doi: 10.1186/s12974-014-0189-0.

El-Ansary, A. K., Bacha, A. Ben & Ayahdi, L. Y. A. (2011). 'Relationship between chronic lead toxicity and plasma neurotransmitters in autistic patients from Saudi Arabia', *Clinical Biochemistry*, *44*(13), pp. 1116–1120. doi: 10.1016/j.clinbiochem.2011.06.982.

Evans, C., et al. (2008). 'Altered amino acid excretion in children with autism', *Nutritional Neuroscience*, *11*(1), pp. 9–17. doi: 10.1179/147683008X301360.

Fatemi, S. H., et al. (2002). 'Glutamic acid decarboxylase 65 and 67 kDa proteins are reduced in autistic parietal and cerebellar cortices', *Biological Psychiatry*, *52*(8), pp. 805–810. doi: 10.1016/S0006-3223(02)01430-0.

Fatemi, S. H. (2008). 'The hyperglutamatergic hypothesis of autism', *Progress in Neuro-Psychopharmacology and Biological Psychiatry*, *32*(3), p. 911. doi: 10.1016/j.pnpbp.2007.11.004.

Ford, T. C., Abu-Akel, A. & Crewther, D. P. (2019). 'The association of excitation and inhibition signaling with the relative symptom expression of autism and psychosis-proneness: Implications for psycho-pharmacology', *Progress in Neuro-Psychopharmacology and Biological Psychiatry*, *88*, pp. 235–242. doi: 10.1016/ j.pnpbp.2018.07.024.

Ford, T. C. & Crewther, D. P. (2016). 'A comprehensive review of the 1H-MRS metabolite spectrum in autism spectrum disorder', *Frontiers in*

*Molecular Neuroscience*, *9*(14), pp. 1–27. doi: 10.3389/fnmol.2016.00014.

Ford, T. C., Nibbs, R. & Crewther, D. P. (2017). 'NeuroImage : Clinical Increased glutamate/GABA + ratio in a shared autistic and schizotypal trait phenotype termed Social Disorganisation', *NeuroImage: Clinical*. Elsevier, *16*(July), pp. 125–131. doi: 10.1016/j.nicl.2017.07.009.

Gabriele, S., Sacco, R. & Persico, A. M. (2014). 'Blood serotonin levels in autism spectrum disorder: A systematic review and', *European Neuropsychopharmacology*. Elsevier, *24*(6), pp. 919–929. doi: 10.1016/j.euroneuro.2014.02.004.

Gaetz, W., et al. (2014). 'NeuroImage GABA estimation in the brains of children on the autism spectrum : Measurement precision and regional cortical variation', *NeuroImage*. Elsevier Inc., *86*, pp. 1–9. doi: 10.1016/j.neuroimage.2013.05.068.

Geier, D. A., et al. (2009). 'A prospective study of transsulfuration biomarkers in autistic disorders', *Neurochemical Research*, *34*(2), p. 394. doi: 10.1007/s11064-008-9888-1.

Ghanizadeh, A. (2013). 'Increased glutamate and homocysteine and decreased glutamine levels in autism: A review and strategies for future studies of amino acids in autism', *Disease Markers*, *35*(5), pp. 281–286. doi: 10.1155/2013/536521.

Good, P. (2011). 'Do salt cravings in children with autistic disorders reveal low blood sodium depleting brain taurine and glutamine ?', *Medical Hypotheses*. Elsevier Ltd, *77*(6), pp. 1015–1021. doi: 10.1016/ j.mehy.2011.08.038.

Guastella, A. J., et al. (2010). 'Intranasal Oxytocin Improves Emotion Recognition for Youth with Autism Spectrum Disorders', *BPS*. Elsevier Inc., *67*(7), pp. 692–694. doi: 10.1016/ j.biopsych.2009.09.020.

Ha, S., et al. (2015). 'Characteristics of Brains in Autism Spectrum Disorder: Structure, Function and Connectivity across the Lifespan', *Experimental Neurobiology*, *24*(4), p. 273. doi: 10.5607/ en.2015.24.4.273.

Hall, M. H., et al. (2015). 'Frontal P3 event-related potential is related to brain glutamine/glutamate ratio measured *in vivo*', *NeuroImage*.

Elsevier Inc., *111*, pp. 186–191. doi: 10.1016/ j.neuroimage. 2015.02.014.

Harada, M., et al. (2011). 'Non-invasive evaluation of the GABAergic/ glutamatergic system in autistic patients observed by MEGA-editing proton MR spectroscopy using a clinical 3 Tesla instrument', *Journal of Autism and Developmental Disorders*, *41*(4), pp. 447–454. doi: 10.1007/s10803-010-1065-0.

Harel-Gadassi, A., et al. (2018). 'Risk for ASD in Preterm Infants: A Three-Year Follow-Up Study', *Autism Research and Treatment*, 2018, pp. 1–9. doi: 10.1155/2018/8316212.

Hassan, T. H., et al. (2013). 'Blood and brain glutamate levels in children with autistic disorder', *Research in Autism Spectrum Disorders*. Elsevier Ltd, *7*(4), pp. 541–548. doi: 10.1016/j.rasd.2012.12.005.

Hesse, S. & Mezger, M. (1978). 'Studies on the mechanism of irreversible protein-binding of aromatic hydrocarbons, mediated by rat liver microsomes: binding of 14C-naphthalene and 14C-1-naphthol', *Naunyn-Schmiedeberg's Archives of Pharmacology*, *354*, pp. 1155–1163. doi: 10.1007/978-3-662-39532-5_91.

Hill, S. D., et al. (1977). 'Diurnal cortisol and temperature variation of normal and autistic children', *Developmental Psychobiology*, *10*(6), pp. 579–583. doi: 10.1002/dev.420100612.

Hisaoka, S., et al. (2001). 'Regional magnetic resonance spectroscopy of the brain in autistic individuals', *Neuroradiology*, *43*(6), pp. 496–498. doi: 10.1007/s002340000520.

Hoffmann, M. (2013). 'The Human Frontal Lobes and Frontal Network Systems: An Evolutionary, Clinical, and Treatment Perspective', *ISRN Neurology*, *2013*(892459), pp. 1–34. doi: 10.1155/2013/892459.

Horder, J., et al. (2013). 'Reduced subcortical glutamate/glutamine in adults with autism spectrum disorders: A [1H]MRS study', *Translational Psychiatry*, *3*(e279), pp. 7–9. doi: 10.1038/tp.2013.53.

Hranilovic, D., et al. (2007). 'Hyperserotonemia in Adults with Autistic Disorder', *J Autism Dev Disord*, *37*, pp. 1934–1940. doi: 10.1007/s10803-006-0324-6.

Husarova, V. M., et al. (2016). 'Plasma oxytocin in children with autism and its correlations with behavioral parameters in children and parents', *Psychiatry Investigation*, *13*(2), pp. 174–183. doi: 10.4306/pi.2016.13.2.174.

Hussman, J. P. (2001). 'Suppresed GABAergic inhibition as a common factor in suspected etiologies of autism', *Journal of Autism and Developmental Disorders*, *31*(2), pp. 247–248.

Joshi, G., et al. (2013). 'Magnetic resonance spectroscopy study of the glutamatergic system in adolescent males with high-functioning autistic disorder: A pilot study at 4T', *European Archives of Psychiatry and Clinical Neuroscience*, *263*(5), pp. 379–384. doi: 10.1007/s00406-012-0369-9.

Kałuzna-Czaplińska, J., et al. (2014). 'Identification of organic acids as potential biomarkers in the urine of autistic children using gas chromatography/mass spectrometry', *Journal of Chromatography B: Analytical Technologies in the Biomedical and Life Sciences*, *966*, pp. 70–76. doi: 10.1016/j.jchromb.2014.01.041.

Kern, J. K., et al. (2011). 'A clinical trial of glutathione supplementation in autism spectrum disorders', *Medical Science Monitor*, *17*(12), pp. 677–682. doi: 10.12659/MSM.882125.

Klausberger, T. & Somogyi, P. (2008). 'Neuronal diversity and temporal dynamics: The unity of hippocampal circuit operations', *Science*, *321*(5885), pp. 53–57. doi: 10.1126/science.1149381.

Kleinhans, N. M., et al. (2007). 'N-acetyl aspartate in autism spectrum disorders: Regional effects and relationship to fMRI activation', *Brain Research*, *1162*(1), pp. 85–97. doi: 10.1016/j.brainres.2007.04.081.

Kobylinska, L., et al. (2019). 'Plasmatic levels of neuropeptides, including oxytocin, in children with autism spectrum disorder, correlate with the disorder severity', *General Endocrinology*, *XV*(11), pp. 16–24. doi: 10.4183/aeb.2019.16.

Kolevzon, A., et al. (2010). 'Relationship between whole blood serotonin and repetitive behaviors in autism', *Psychiatry Research*. Elsevier Ltd, *175*(3), pp. 274–276. doi: 10.1016/j.psychres.2009.02.008.

Van Kooten, I. A. J., Hof, P. R. & Engeland, H. Van (2005). 'Autism: Neuropathology, alterations of the GABAergic system, and animal models', *International Review of Neurobiology*, *71*(05), pp. 1–26. doi: 10.1016/S0074-7742(05)71001-1.

Kuwabara, H., et al. (2013). 'Altered Metabolites in the Plasma of Autism Spectrum Disorder: A Capillary Electrophoresis Time-of-Flight Mass Spectroscopy Study', *PLoS ONE*, *8*(9). doi: 10.1371/ journal. pone.0073814.

Lam, K. S. L., Aman, M. G. & Arnold, L. E. (2006). 'Neurochemical correlates of autistic disorder: A review of the literature', *Research in Developmental Disabilities*, *27*(3), pp. 254–289. doi: 10.1016/ j.ridd.2005.03.003.

Lodge, D. (2009). 'The history of the pharmacology and cloning of ionotropic glutamate receptors and the development of idiosyncratic nomenclature', *Neuropharmacology*. Elsevier Ltd, *56*(1), pp. 6–21. doi: 10.1016/j.neuropharm.2008.08.006.

Lopatina, O. L., et al. (2018). 'Oxytocin and excitation/inhibition balance in social recognition', *Neuropeptides*. Elsevier Ltd, *72*, pp. 1–11. doi: 10.1016/j.npep.2018.09.003.

Lv, J. & Liu, F. (2017). 'The role of serotonin beyond the central nervous system during embryogenesis', *Frontiers in Cellular Neuroscience*, *11*(74), pp. 1–7. doi: 10.3389/fncel.2017.00074.

Manent, J. B. & Represa, A. (2007). 'Neurotransmitters and brain maturation: Early paracrine actions of GABA and glutamate modulate neuronal migration', *Neuroscientist*, *13*(3), pp. 268–279. doi: 10.1177/1073858406298918.

Martin, E. R., et al. (2000). 'Analysis of linkage disequilibrium in γ-aminobutyric acid receptor subunit genes in autistic disorder', *American Journal of Medical Genetics - Neuropsychiatric Genetics*, *96*(1), pp. 43–48. doi: 10.1002/(SICI)1096-8628(20000207)96: 1<43::AID-AJMG9>3.0.CO;2-3.

Di Martino, A., et al. (2008). 'Functional Brain Correlates of Social and Nonsocial Processes in Autism Spectrum Disorders : An Activation

Likelihood Estimation Meta-Analysis', *BPS. Society of Biological Psychiatry*, *65*(1), pp. 63–74. doi: 10.1016/j.biopsych.2008.09.022.

Mcbride, P. A., et al. (1988). 'Serotonergic Responsivity in Male Young Adults With Autistic Disorder', *Arch Gen Psychiatry*, *46*, pp. 213–221.

Ming, X., et al. (2012). 'Metabolic perturbance in autism spectrum disorders: A metabolomics study', *Journal of Proteome Research*, *11*(12), pp. 5856–5862. doi: 10.1021/pr300910n.

Modahl, C., et al. (1998). 'Plasma oxytocin levels in autistic children', *Biological Psychiatry*, *43*(4), pp. 270–277. doi: 10.1016/S0006-3223(97)00439-3.

Moffett, J. R., et al. (2007). 'N-Acetylaspartate in the CNS: From neurodiagnostics to neurobiology', *Progress in Neurobiology*, *81*(2), pp. 89–131. doi: 10.1016/j.pneurobio.2006.12.003.

Moreno-Fuenmayor, H., Borjas, L., Arrieta, A. & Valera, V. S. C. L. (1996). 'Plasma excitatory amino acids in autism', *Investigacion Clinica*, *37*(2), pp. 113–128.

Mück-Seler, D. & Pivac, N. (2011). 'Serotonin', *Periodicum Biologorum*, *113*(1), pp. 29–41.

Muller, C. L. & Anacker, A. M. J. (2015). 'The serotonin system in autism spectrum disorder: from biomarker to animal models', *Neuroscience*, *321*, pp. 24–41. doi: 10.1016/j.neuroscience.2015.11.010.

Nadal-Desbarats, L., et al. (2014). 'Combined 1H-NMR and 1H–13C HSQC-NMR to improve urinary screening in autism spectrum disorders', *Analyst*, *139*, pp. 3460–3468. doi: 10.1039/c4an00552j.

Naushad, S. M., et al. (2013). 'Autistic children exhibit distinct plasma amino acid profile', *Indian Journal of Biochemistry and Biophysics*, *50*(5), pp. 474–478.

Noto, A., et al. (2014). 'The urinary metabolomics profile of an Italian autistic children population and their unaffected siblings', *Journal of Maternal-Fetal and Neonatal Medicine*, *27*(52), pp. 46–52. doi: 10.3109/14767058.2014.954784.

Öngür, D., et al. (2009). 'Abnormal glutamatergic neurotransmission and neuronalglial interactions in acute mania', *Biol Psychiatry*, *64*(8), pp. 718–726. doi: 10.1016/j.biopsych.2008.05.014.

Ortinski, P. I., et al. (2010). 'Selective induction of astrocytic gliosis generates deficits in neuronal inhibition', *Nature Neuroscience*, *13*(5), pp. 584–591. doi: 10.1038/nn.2535.

Owens, D. F. & Kriegstein, A. R. (2002). 'Is there more to GABA than synaptic inhibition?', *Nature Reviews Neuroscience*, pp. 715–727. doi: 10.1038/nrn919.

Page, L. A., et al. (2006). '*In vivo* 1H-magnetic resonance spectroscopy study of amygdala-hippocampal and parietal regions in autism', *American Journal of Psychiatry*, *163*(12), pp. 2189–2192. doi: 10.1176/ajp.2006.163.12.2189.

Palmen, S. J. M. C., et al. (2004). 'Neuropathological findings in autism', *Brain*, *127*(12), pp. 2572–2583. doi: 10.1093/brain/awh287.

Park, E. & Cohen, I. (2017). 'Is Taurine a Biomarker in Autistic Spectrum Disorder?', *Advances in Experimental Medicine and Biology*, *975*, pp. 551–561. doi: 10.1007/978-94-024-1079-2.

Patrick, R. P. & Ames, B. N. (2014). 'Vitamin D hormone regulates serotonin synthesis . Part 1 : relevance for autism', *The FASEB Journal*, *28*(6), pp. 2398–2413. doi: 10.1096/fj.13-246546.

Pereira, F. C., et al. (2008). 'Acute increase of the glutamate-glutamine cycling in discrete brain areas after administration of a single dose of amphetamine', in *Annals of the New York Academy of Sciences*, pp. 212–221. doi: 10.1196/annals.1432.040.

Pietraszek, M. H., et al. (1992). 'Relationship between serotonergic measures in periphery and the brain of mouse', *Life Sciences*, *51*(1), pp. 75–82.

Pizzarelli, R. & Cherubini, E. (2011). 'Alterations of GABAergic signaling in autism spectrum disorders', *Neural Plasticity*, *2011*(297153), pp. 1–12. doi: 10.1155/2011/297153.

Puts, N. A. J., et al. (2017). 'Reduced GABA and Altered Somatosensory Function in Children with Autism Spectrum Disorder', *Autism Res.*, *10*(4), pp. 608–619. doi: 10.1002/aur.1691.

Rajmohan, V. & Mohandas, E. (2019). 'The limbic system', *Indian J Psychiatry.*, *49*(2), pp. 132–139.

Rojas, D. C., et al. (2014). 'Decreased left perisylvian GABA concentration in children with autism and unaffected siblings', *NeuroImage*. Elsevier Inc., *86*, pp. 28–34. doi: 10.1016/j.neuroimage.2013.01.045.

Rolf, L., et al. (1993). 'Serotonin and amino acid content in platelets of autistic children', *Actu Psychiutr Scund*, *87*, pp. 312–316.

Rosenberg, A., Patterson, J. S. & Angelaki, D. E. (2015). 'A computational perspective on autism', *Proceedings of the National Academy of Sciences of the United States of America*, *112*(30), pp. 9158–9165. doi: 10.1073/pnas.1510583112.

Rutigliano, G., et al. (2016). 'Peripheral oxytocin and vasopressin: Biomarkers of psychiatric disorders? A comprehensive systematic review and preliminary meta-analysis', *Psychiatry Research*, *241*, pp. 207–220. doi: 10.1016/j.psychres.2016.04.117.

Sacrey, L. A. R., Bennett, J. A. & Zwaigenbaum, L. (2015). 'Early Infant Development and Intervention for Autism Spectrum Disorder', *Journal of Child Neurology*, *30*(14), pp. 1921–1929. doi: 10.1177/08830 73815601500.

Sheldon, A. L. & Robinson, M. B. (2008). 'Diseases and Potential Opportunities for Intervention', *Pediatrics*, *51*(215), pp. 333–355.

Shimmura, C., et al. (2011). 'Alteration of plasma glutamate and glutamine levels in children with high-functioning autism', *PLoS ONE*, *6*(10), pp. 2–7. doi: 10.1371/journal.pone.0025340.

Shimmura, C., et al. (2013). 'Enzymes in the glutamate-glutamine cycle in the anterior cingulate cortex in postmortem brain of subjects with autism', *Molecular Autism*, *4*(6), pp. 1–7. doi: 10.1186/2040-2392-4-6.

Shinohe, A., et al. (2006). 'Increased serum levels of glutamate in adult patients with autism', *Progress in Neuro-Psychopharmacology and Biological Psychiatry*, *30*(8), pp. 1472–1477. doi: 10.1016/j.pnpbp.2006.06.013.

Sibilla, S. & Ballerini, L. (2009). 'GABAergic and glycinergic interneuron expression during spinal cord development: Dynamic interplay between inhibition and excitation in the control of ventral network outputs', *Progress in Neurobiology*, *89*(1), pp. 46–60. doi: 10.1016/j.pneurobio.2009.06.001.

Stelmashook, E. V., et al. (2011). 'Role of glutamine in neuronal survival and death during brain ischemia and hypoglycemia', *International Journal of Neuroscience*, *121*(8), pp. 415–422. doi: 10.3109/00207454.2011.570464.

Tan, Y., et al. (2019). 'Oxytocin receptors are expressed by glutamatergic prefrontal cortical neurons that selectively modulate social recognition modulate social recognition Abbreviated title : Oxytocin receptors and social recognition . Affiliations : 1 Department of Pharmacod', *J Neurosci*, *39*(17), pp. 3249–3263. doi: 10.1523/JNEUROSCI.2944-18.2019.

Tanaka, M., et al. (2018). 'Brain hyperserotonemia causes autism-relevant social deficits in mice', *Molecular Autism*, *9*(1), pp. 1–14. doi: 10.1186/s13229-018-0243-3.

Tapiero, H., et al. (2002). 'II. Glutamine and glutamate', *Biomed Pharmacother*, *56*, 56, pp. 446–457.

Tekin, S. & Cummings, J. L. (2002). 'Frontal-subcortical neuronal circuits and clinical neuropsychiatry: An update', *Journal of Psychosomatic Research*, *53*(2), pp. 647–654. doi: 10.1016/S0022-3999(02)00428-2.

Tirouvanziam, Rabindra Obukhanych, Tetyana V. Laval, J., et al. (2012). 'Distinct Plasma Profile of Polar Neutral Amino Acids, Leucine, and Glutamate in Children with Autism Spectrum Disorders', *J Autism Dev Disord*, *42*, pp. 827–836. doi: 10.1007/s10803-011-1314-x.

Tordjman, S., et al. (1997). 'Plasma beta-endorphin, adrenocorticotropin hormone, and cortisol in autism.', *Journal of child psychology and psychiatry, and allied disciplines*, *38*(6), pp. 705–715.

Tu, W. J., Chen, H. & He, J. (2012). 'Application of LC-MS/MS analysis of plasma amino acids profiles in children with autism', *J. Clin. Biochem. Nutr.*, 51(3), pp. 248–249. doi: 10.3164/jcbn.

U.S. Department of Health and Human Services. (2012). *Prevalence of Autism Spectrum Disorders — Autism and Developmental Disabilities Monitoring Network,* 14 Sites, United States, 2008, MMWR Surveill Summ.

Voinsky, I., et al. (2019). 'Peripheral Blood Mononuclear Cell Oxytocin and Vasopressin Receptor Expression Positively Correlates with Social and

Behavioral Function in Children with Autism', *Scientific Reports*, *9*(13443), pp. 1–10. doi: 10.1038/s41598-019-49617-9.

Walsh, P., et al. (2011). 'In search of biomarkers for autism: scientific, social and ethical challenges', *Nat Rev Neurosci*, *12*(10), pp. 603–612.

Wan, M. W., et al. (2013). 'Quality of interaction between at-risk infants and caregiver at 12-15 months is associated with 3-year autism outcome', *Journal of Child Psychology and Psychiatry and Allied Disciplines*, *54*(7), pp. 763–771. doi: 10.1111/jcpp.12032.

Won, H., et al. (2012). 'Autistic-like social behaviour in Shank2-mutant mice improved by restoring NMDA receptor function', *Nature*, *486*(7402), pp. 261–265. doi: 10.1038/nature11208.

Yap, I. K. S., et al. (2010). 'Urinary Metabolic Phenotyping Differentiates Children with Autism from Their Unaffected Siblings and Age-Matched Controls', *Journal of Proteome Research*, *9*, pp. 2996–3004.

Yüksel, C. & Öngür, D. (2010). 'Magnetic Resonance Spectroscopy Studies of Glutamate-Related Abnormalities in Mood Disorders', *BPS*. Elsevier Inc., *68*(9), pp. 785–794. doi: 10.1016/ j.biopsych.2010.06.016.

Zhang, B., et al. (2018). 'Central insulin action induces activation of paraventricular oxytocin neurons to release oxytocin into circulation', *Scientific Reports*, *8*(1), pp. 1–5. doi: 10.1038/s41598-018-28816-w.

Zheng, H. F., et al. (2017). 'Body fluid levels of neuroactive amino acids in autism spectrum disorders: a review of the literature', *Amino Acids*, pp. 57–65. doi: 10.1007/s00726-016-2332-y.

Zheng, Z., et al. (2016). 'Blood glutamate levels in autism spectrum disorder: A systematic review and meta-analysis', *PLoS ONE*, *11*(7), pp. 2–13. doi: 10.1371/journal.pone.0158688.

Zwaigenbaum, L., et al. (2016). 'Stability of diagnostic assessment for autism spectrum disorder between 18 and 36 months in a high-risk cohort', *Autism Research*, *9*(7), pp. 790–800. doi: 10.1002/aur.1585.

In: Understanding Children with Autism … ISBN: 978-1-53617-647-6
Editor: Anne Bourque 

*Chapter 6*

# The Experience of Embarrassment in Children with Autism Spectrum Disorders

***Denise Davidson[1], Juhi Lilwani[2], Kyra Zagorski[1], Kaitlyn Foust[1] and Bridget Melody[1]***

[1]Department of Psychology, Loyola University Chicago, Chicago, IL, US

[2]Department of Counseling Psychology, Loyola University Chicago, Chicago, IL, US

## Abstract

Factors that contribute to the complexity of the emotion of embarrassment were studied in this research. Twenty-three children with Autism Spectrum Disorders (ASD) and 25 neurotypical children were asked to complete an embarrassment measure that tapped into three faucets of their understanding of embarrassment. Specifically, we examined whether children were aware of the role of the audience when asked to imagine themselves in embarrassing situations, whether they were able to distinguish between intense and mildly embarrassing situations happening to another child, and the extent to which children could recount their own embarrassing experiences. Additionally, this study assessed the relations between ASD symptomatology, theory of mind (ToM), and other individual factors (FSIQ, age) on children's responses across the embarrassment tasks. When asked to imagine themselves in an embarrassing situation, all of the children labeled the active (derisive) audience vignette to be the most embarrassing and the vignette with no audience to be the least embarrassing. However, children with ASD were significantly more likely to find the passive audience (i.e., an audience is present but makes no comment) vignette to be embarrassing. Children with ASD were also less accurate in identifying and recounting embarrassing situations than neurotypical children. Greater ToM ability was correlated with a better understanding of embarrassment in children with ASD, especially when asked to imagine themselves in an embarrassing scenario with a derisive audience present. Greater ASD symptomatology was also correlated with a less accurate understanding of embarrassment in this same condition. The present study's implications and future research directions are discussed.

**Keywords:** autism, emotion, embarrassment, theory of mind, children

# INTRODUCTION

## Overview: Characteristics and Functions of Embarrassment

According to Miller (2007), "embarrassment is an acute state of startled, flustered abashment and chagrin that results from events that increase the threat of unwanted evaluations from real or imagined audiences" (p. 246). Most embarrassing acts involve the violation of social or cultural norms, missteps or mishaps, or perceived appearance flaws. Embarrassment is often a subjective experience, with individuals reporting that they felt scrutinized by others regardless of whether this was the case. In fact, the degree to which an individual experiences embarrassment is not always commensurate with the actual event. This phenomenon is referred to as the "spotlight effect," or the tendency to assume that our actions are more salient and important to others than they really are (Gilovioch, Medvec, & Savitsky, 2000). Thus, the experience of embarrassment can be quite anxiety-provoking for some individuals, and "even lead to clinical disorders in some cases" (p. 1; Feinberg, Willer, & Keltner, 2011).

Nevertheless, scholars believe that the experience of embarrassment, although typically a negative emotional state, serves a number of purposes. Miller (1996; 2007), as well as others (Feinberg et al., 2011; Goffman, 1956), suggest that embarrassment evolved as a way to maintain social order. For example, by displaying signs of embarrassment after committing an embarrassing act, people communicate to others that they recognize and regret their mistake. For highly egregious acts such as committing a crime, the perception of getting caught and the subsequent embarrassment felt helps serve as a deterrent, benefitting both society and the individual. According to Keltner and Buswell (1997), "people's experience and display of embarrassment, from this perspective, play a critical role in socialization practices, such as teasing and punishment, the motivation of moral behavior and conformity, the development of the conscience, and the negotiation of social roles and status" (p. 250). Embarrassment can serve us in more subtle ways too, as it may elicit from others kindly, supportive reactions that help us quickly overcome our missteps.

Over the years, scholars have tried to illuminate the defining characteristics of embarrassment. Most, if not all, agree that embarrass-ment is a complex, self-conscious emotion (Tracy & Robins, 2007). Self-conscious emotions are a special class of emotions that require self-awareness and self-representation, which in turn enables one to engage in self-evaluation, a process that is essential for experiencing embarrassment (Tracy & Robins, 2007). Although sharing properties with other self-conscious emotions (e.g., shame, guilt), a number of studies have found that embarrassment is a unique emotion that can be distinguished, at least in part, from other self-conscious emotions by its antecedents (Keltner & Buswell, 1997). To illustrate, shame follows the failure to live up to expectations that define the core or global self, such as failing to live up to one's personal or moral ideals, whereas guilt usually follows from individual transgressions of moral rules (e.g., lying, cheating). In contrast, the antecedents of embarrassment often arise from transgressions of social conventions, including physical mishaps (e.g., tripping), losing self-control (e.g., belching), cognitive shortcomings (e.g., forgetting another's name), or losing privacy regarding personal issues. In fact, the link between embarrassment and social conventions may explain why embarrassment tends to be experienced less intensely among family and friends than among strangers (Keltner & Buswell, 1997).

## Development of Embarrassment in Neurotypical and Neurodiverse (ASD) Children

At least one study has shown that the expression of embarrassment can be seen as early as infancy in neurotypical children (Reddy, 2000). However, the ability to attribute embarrassment to others and to oneself appears to develop later during childhood (e.g., Bennett, 1989; Bennett & Gillingham, 1991; Bennett, Yuill, Banerjess, & Thompson, 1998). In Bennett's (1989) study, children between 5 and 13 years of age were presented with hypothetical scenarios that involved no audience, a passive audience, or an active (derisive) audience. Children were asked to report how they would feel if the event happened to them and why. Results showed that the 5- and 8-year-old children reported embarrassment in the active audience condition, whereas older children reported embarrassment in the active and passive audience conditions.

In later research, Colonesi, Englehard, and Bögels (2010) provided 4- to 9-year-old neurotypical children with brief stories in which the main character received negative, positive or neutral social reactions. Using verbal, free response measures, older children reported more embarrassment in the negative and neutral conditions than younger children, although no age-related differences were found in the non-verbal condition (i.e., children pointed to faces expressing different emotions including embarrassment). In Colonesi et al.'s (2010) study, they found that theory of mind (ToM) understanding, or individuals' ability to take the perspective of others, was not related to children's attributions of embarrassment. However, only "first-level" understanding of false beliefs—a measure of ToM, was examined in their study. It may be that a different picture emerges between ToM ability and attributions of embarrassment when evaluating first- and more advanced, second-order false belief understanding.

In early research comparing children with and without ASD, Capps, Yirmiya, and Sigman (1992) asked children to think of and share an example of when they experienced several emotions (i.e., happiness, sadness, pride, and embarrassment). Children were also asked to label the different emotional states a child displayed in eight photographs. Children with ASD differed from neurotypical children most significantly in their descriptions of embarrassment. Specifically, children with ASD reported external and uncontrollable events for embarrassment, differing from the neurotypical responses for embarrassment which described internal and controllable events. Furthermore, children with ASD reported significantly less instances of embarrassment that occurred in the presence of an audience. The authors suggested that this finding demonstrates that children with ASD have a more limited understanding of embarrassment. Additionally, children with ASD also required more time to produce answers and needed more prompting, thereby demonstrating the challenge understanding embarrassment presented.

Determined to test whether children with ASD do in fact experience embarrassment in different situations, Hillier and Allinson (2002a) conducted a second study where participants were presented with either non-embarrassing, embarrassing, or imagined embarrassing situations and asked to rate the level of embarrassment the main character in the situation felt and to provide justification for their answers. Hillier and Allinson (2002a) assessed four different groups of children: children with ASD, children with learning difficulties, younger neurotypical children and older neurotypical children. Children rated the level of embarrassment by selecting one of three schematic faces which represented the responses of "not at all embarrassed," "quite embarrassed," and "very embarrassed." Hillier and Allinson (2002a) predicted that participants who had showed well-developed ToM ability would perform the most accurately and provide the most sound justifications.

The results revealed that children with ASD demonstrated a better understanding of embarrassment than was predicted, but still lacked a complex understanding of the emotion. For example, children with ASD did not rate the imagined embarrassing scenarios as significantly less embarrassing than the embarrassing scenarios, and children with ASD showed less ability to differentiate scenarios that should cause embarrassment from scenarios that should not. Children with ASD also struggled with providing appropriate justifications for why the main character would feel or not feel embarrassed in embarrassing and non-embarrassing scenarios. According to the authors, an understanding of embarrassment may lack complexity and depth for children with autism.

In another study by Hillier and Allinson (2002b), the authors provided more optimistic findings in regard to understanding of embarrassment in ASD. In this study, Hillier and Allinson (2002b) used a participant pool and procedure that was similar to their first study, except that they measured the level of embarrassment children would feel depending on whether an audience was present, the type of audience present (i.e., a best friend or authority figure), and whether or not the main character thought he/she had been seen. The authors found that there were no significant differences between children with ASD and neurotypical children in their identification of embarrassing scenarios when an audience was present, as all children rated the scenarios more embarrassing when witnessed by an audience. Similarly, children with ASD and neurotypical younger children both rated scenarios where an authority figure witnessed a faux pas to be more embarrassing than scenarios where a best friend witnessed a faux pas. Nevertheless, the authors found that children with ASD struggled with accurately justifying their ratings of embarrassment. Children with ASD also struggled with an empathy scenario, which the authors suggested demonstrated their difficulty in understanding the mental states of others due to challenges with ToM (Hillier & Allinson, 2002b).

## Mechanisms Underlying Embarrassment Understanding

In addition to ToM, other mechanisms may underlie children's understanding of embarrassment. Thus, a goal of the present research was to examine several potential mechanisms that underlie children's responses on embarrassment measures, including ASD symptomatology, ToM, full-scale IQ (FSIQ) and age. ASD symptomology, such as social responsiveness, may affect one's understanding of the nuances of embarrassment. Given that embarrassment is a highly social emotion that has important roots in social relations and its conventions, it may be that social responsiveness is related to children's understanding of the complexities of embarrassment. Although research on basic emotion processing has shown that difficulties with social responsiveness were related to errors on emotion recognition tests (Tell, Davidson, & Camras, 2014), and were associated with atypical eye gaze patterns when processing dynamic social and emotional scenes for children with ASD (Speer, Cook, McMahon, & Clark, 2007), it is not known how ASD symptomatology affects one's understanding of embarrassment.

We were also interested in examining the relations between ToM and children's understanding of embarrassment. According to Nader-Grosbois and Day (2011), ToM reflects one's ability to understand the mental states of others, such as the desires and intentions of others. It also enables one to better understand one's own mind and mental state. Past research has shown that ToM skills were positively associated with the ability to recognize basic emotions from faces (Tell et al., 2014). However, while a number of past studies have suggested that there is an association between ToM ability and an understanding of embarrassment, not all studies have empirically assessed this relation. Finally, we explored whether FSIQ and age were related to children's responses across our embarrassment tasks. To our knowledge, past studies have not explored the associations between these variables and children's understanding of embarrassment.

## The Present Study

In the present study, 9- to 14-year-old children with and without ASD matched on a number of variables (see Table 1) were asked to complete an embarrassment measure that consisted of three different tasks designed to capture various aspects of children's understanding of embarrassment in themselves and in others. The first task assessed children's understanding of the role of the audience in the experience of embarrassment by asking them to imagine themselves in the scenarios. In the second task, children were asked to identify embarrassing situations from a number of emotional events using vignettes that reflected intensely and less intensely events. For this task, children were asked to identify when a protagonist would feel embarrassed. In the third task, children were asked to recount two personal experiences of embarrassment. A number of variables were assessed in their recounts including, but not limited to, the appropriateness of their content, whether they used causal inferences, the number of prompts needed to elicit two recounts, and whether they mentioned a violation of a social convention in their recounts. Lastly, we assessed the extent to which ASD symptomatology, ToM ability and other individual factors (FSIQ, age) affected children's performance across the three tasks.

Research questions were as follows:

1. Firstly, are children with and without ASD equally aware of the role of the audience in embarrassing situations? Are both groups able to distinguish between no audience being present, a passive audience that provides no judgment of the embarrassing act, and an active audience that provides negative judgment (e.g., laughter, teasing) when asked to imagine themselves in the situation?
2. Secondly, are children with and without ASD equally capable of distinguishing embarrassing situations from other emotion-provoking situations, and are they capable of distinguishing between intense and less intense examples of embarrassing situations? Do they understand that some situations may be more intense and produce a more lasting experience of the emotion?

3. Finally, are children with and without ASD similar in their recounting of experiences of embarrassment? Using linguistic analyses, we examined a number of variables in their recounts, as noted above. Studies have shown that children with ASD struggle with recounting more complex emotions, may provide less appropriate content, and may need more prompting to elicit the recount for complex emotions but not basic emotions (Losh & Capps, 2006). However, past research did not isolate the types of complex emotions and did not focus specifically on embarrassment.

# METHODS

## Participants

A total of 48 children participated in the research study: 23 children with ASD, which included 19 males and 4 females ($M_{age}$ = 11;10, Range = 7;09 – 14;06), and 25 neurotypical children, 19 males and 6 females ($M_{age}$ = 11;08, Range = 8;02 – 14;05). Consistent with previous research on emotion processing in children with ASD (e.g., Begeer, Reiffe, Terwogt, & Stockmann, 2006; Davidson, Hilvert, Misiunaite, & Giordano, 2018; Tell & Davidson, 2014), a broad age range was used in order to assess the association between age and children's understanding of embarrassment across several measures. To be eligible for participation, all children had to have an overall IQ of $\geq$ 70 as determined by the Wechsler Abbreviated Scale of Intelligence, Second Edition (WASI-II; Wechsler, 2011), and be native speakers of English as reported by their parents. All children were recruited from a school district in a middle-class suburb of a large urban city in the United States. Additional participant characteristics are provided in Table 1.

**Table 1. Participant Characteristics of Children with ASD and Neurotypical (NT) Children**

| | NT ($n$ = 25) | ASD ($n$ = 23) |
|---|---|---|
| | Mean (SD) | |
| Age | 11;10 (2;01) | 11;06 (2;02) |
| Male:Female | 19:5 | 19:5 |
| Full-Scale IQ | 107.72 (12.21)[a] | 96.65 (18.99) |
| SRS-2 T-Score | 47.32 (7.19)[a] | 74.09 (8.68) |
| SRS-2 Severity Group | | |
| Normal (59 and below) | 24 | 0 |
| Mild (60-65) | 0 | 3 |
| Moderate (66-75) | 0 | 12 |
| Severe (76 or higher) | 0 | 8 |
| CARS-2 T-Score | -- | 46.52 (6.19) |
| CARS-2 Severity Group | | |
| Mild-to-Moderate | -- | 18 |
| Severe | -- | 5 |
| Faux Pas Detection Score | 6.08 (2.53) | 5.22 (3.12) |
| SCQ | 3.41 (3.41)[a] | 21.21 (5.69) |

*Note.* SRS-2 = Social Responsiveness Scale, Second Edition. CARS-2 = Childhood Autism Rating Scale, Second Edition. SCQ = Social Communication Questionnaire. [a] Significant difference between NT and ASD children.

### *Children with ASD*

All children with ASD were receiving services in their schools under an autism classification that was established through a multidisciplinary evaluation. In order to receive these services, clinical diagnosis of children with ASD had been determined by a pediatrician or a licensed psychologist in accordance with the *Diagnostic and Statistical Manual of Mental Disorders-IV* or *V* (APA, 2000; 2013). ASD symptom severity was established through the Childhood Autism Rating Scale, Second Edition (CARS-2; Schopler, Van Bourgondien, Wellman, & Love, 2010), the Social Responsiveness Scale, Second Edition (SRS-2; Constantino, 2012), and the Social Communication Questionnaire (SCQ; Rutter, Bailey, & Lord 2003).

The CARS-2 assists in the identification of children with ASD and determines symptom severity through a 15-item behavior rating scale that is based on direct observation by the examiner as well as parent report. The CARS-2 shows strong interrater reliability (.95), high internal consistency (.96), and good concurrent validity (.77) with the Autism Diagnostic Observation Schedule (ADOS; Lord & Corsello, 2005). All children with ASD received an overall score that placed them in the mild-to-moderate ($N = 18$) or severe ($N = 5$) symptomatology group (see Table 1).

The presence and severity of social impairment associated with ASD was established through the use of the SRS-2, a 65-item parent questionnaire. The SRS-2 shows good interrater reliability (r = .61 - .92) and high internal consistency ($\alpha = .95$). Mean total scores (T-scores) are given in Table 1. Scores on the SRS-2 are designed to be in line with the ASD diagnostic criteria of the DSM (Constantino & Gruber, 2012). In the present study, five children with ASD were in the mild-range (60 - 65 T-Score), eight were in the moderate range (66 - 75 T-score), and seven were in the severe range (76 T-Score or higher). Three children were missing their parents' SRS-2 questionnaire. However, no differences were found in age, $t(21) = -.87$, $p = .40$, $d = .60$, or CARS-2 T-scores, $t(21) = -.64$, $p = .53$, $d = .34$, between children who had an SRS-2 score and those who did not.

Additionally, ASD-level symptoms were confirmed with the SCQ (Rutter et al., 2003), a 40-item parent questionnaire that asks about children's communication skills and social functioning that are characteristic of ASD. The SCQ has shown good sensitivity (.88) and specificity (.72) with an ASD diagnosis (Chandler et al., 2007). Scores above 15 suggest the individual is likely to have ASD (see Table 1). Seventeen children with ASD scored above 15, and two scored below 15 (i.e., 11, 12). Four parents did not return the SCQ. No significant differences were found in age, $t(20) = -.36$, $p = .73$, $d = .17$, or CARS-2 T-scores, $t(20) = -.30$, $p = .77$, $d = .16$, between children who had an SCQ score and children with ASD who did not.

### *Neurotypical Children*

Parents of neurotypical children also completed the SRS-2 and SCQ to determine that their children did not exhibit significant ASD symptoms. All neurotypical children obtained scores on the SRS-2 and SCQ below the thresholds for ASD-level symptomatology and, as expected, scored significantly lower on both measures compared to children with ASD. See Table 1 for group means and comparisons.

## Measures and Procedure

All materials and procedures were approved before the start of the study by the Institutional Review Board at the host university. Children were tested following parent written consent and verbal consent of the children. The present research was part of a larger study on emotion processing in children with ASD. Children completed all measures in a randomized order.

### *Embarrassment Measures*

Children were presented with an embarrassment measure that consisted of three different assessments of children's understanding of embarrassment. Presentation of the three tasks was randomized across children in each diagnostic group. Vignettes and situations used in the first two tasks were adapted from previous research (e.g., Davidson, 2006).

In the *Audience Awareness* task, children were read brief vignettes describing an everyday emotional situation that was designed to convey a potentially embarrassing situation (see Table 2). Three different types of emotional situations were described. In the Active Audience condition, the child was asked to imagine that he or she committed an embarrassing act in front of an audience (e.g., other children) and was reprimanded or made fun of in some way for the act. In the Passive Audience condition, an audience supposedly witnessed the participant committing the gaffe but did not comment on it in any way. Finally, in the No Audience condition, the participant was asked to imagine committing a potentially embarrassing act without an audience present.

**Table 2. Examples of Audience Awareness Embarrassment Vignettes**

| Condition | Audience Awareness Examples |
|---|---|
| Active Audience | At the school you attend, you eat lunch in the cafeteria every day. Once you get your food, you carry your tray to a table to eat it. Just as you are walking to the table you bump into a chair and you end up dropping your tray of food. Food goes everywhere. The other kids in the cafeteria laugh at you and some point their finger at you. |
| Passive Audience | Your dad decided to take you and your friends to see a movie you really wanted to see. Your dad buys each of you some popcorn and drinks. When you are walking down the aisle to find some good seats, you trip and spill your popcorn all over the place. Your friends see you trip, as does the rest of the people in the movie theater but no one says anything. |
| No Audience | One day you went to the grocery store with your mom. You did not watch where you were going and you ended up knocking over a large display of canned goods. You looked around and noticed that no one else saw you do it and no one was in the aisle. |

At the start of this task, children were told, "I'm going to read you three very short stories and you will be asked to imagine that what happened in the story has happened to you. After hearing each story, I will ask you a few questions about the story. Is that ok?" A story reflecting one of the three conditions was read, and children were asked using a free response format: "How would you feel if that happened to you in real life?" They were then provided with a list of emotion words (i.e., guilty, proud, sad, happy, angry, embarrassed) in a random order and asked to choose one. Next they were asked why they would feel that way, with their answers recorded verbatim. Story conditions were presented in a random order.

In the *Situational Embarrassment* task, children were presented with two embarrassing scenarios, one that was designed to elicit significant embarrassment (Intense Condition) and one that was designed to elicit mild embarrassment (Less Intense Condition), see Table 3. Children were also presented with intense and less intense examples of three basic emotions (i.e., happy, fear, sad), and two additional, self-conscious emotions (i.e., pride, guilt) as part of the larger study, although only children's responses to the embarrassing situations were analyzed for this paper. Using a free response format, children were first asked to label the emotion they thought the protagonist "would be feeling" in the situation. Afterwards, using a forced-choice format, children were given a list of emotion words in a random order (i.e., guilty, proud, sad, happy, angry, embarrassed) and were asked to choose the word from the list that best reflected how the child in the story felt. Children were asked to rate the intensity of the emotion they thought would be elicited by the situation on a scale from 1 to 5 (i.e., "Sometimes you feel an emotion strongly and sometimes you feel it very little. On a scale from 1-5, with 5 being the strongest, I'm going to ask you to tell me how strongly you think the child in the story feels that emotion."), as well as the duration of the emotion on a scale from 1-5, with 5 being "a really long time."

**Table 3. Examples of Situational Embarrassment Vignettes**

| **Picture** | **Situational Embarrassment Examples Vignette** | **Intensity** |
|---|---|---|
| 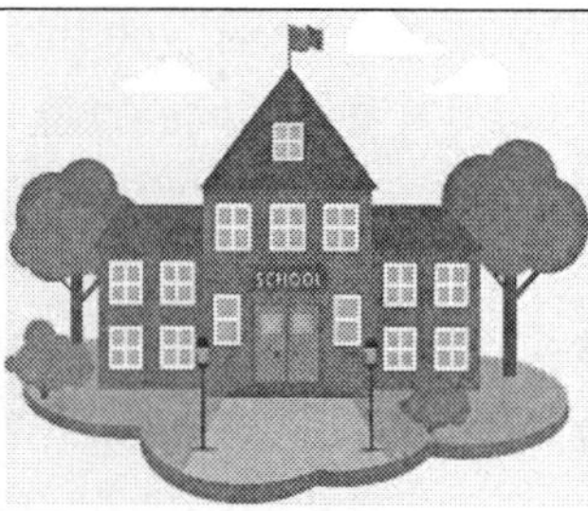 | Maria has been at her new school for just a couple of weeks. The school is very big, with lots of hallways and classrooms. Yesterday, Maria got lost walking in the hallway and could not find her classroom. Maria felt__________ that her new classmates saw her get lost in the hallway. | Low |
| 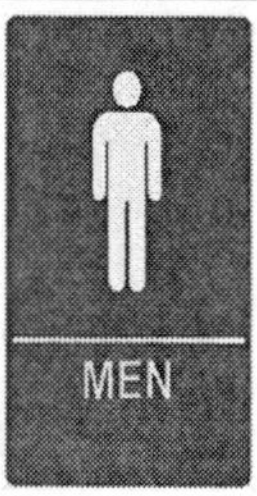  | Maria just started going to a new school. The school is very big, with lots of hallways and classrooms. Yesterday at school, Maria had to go to the bathroom. Unfortunately, Maria wasn't paying attention and she went into the boy's bathroom by mistake. A bunch of boys saw her and started laughing at her. Maria was ________ that the boys saw her and were making fun of her. | High |

Finally, in the *Recounting Embarrassing Situations* task, children were asked to recount two personal experiences or situations that led to embarrassment in themselves as part of a larger task asking children to recount three basic emotional experiences (i.e., happy, fear, sad), and two additional self-conscious emotional experiences (i.e., pride, guilt). In the *Recounting Embarrassing Situations* task children were told, "Now, I'd like for you to tell me about different times when you felt a certain way. For example, if someone asked me to tell them about a time I felt surprised, I would tell them about a time my mom and dad threw me a birthday party when I was 10 years old. I had to stay late after school on my birthday for cheerleading, so we were planning on celebrating on a different day. But then when I came home, I opened the door and lots of my friends and family members were there. They all shouted surprise! It was great because we ate cake and ice cream and I got to open up presents. Because I wasn't expecting anything special, I was really surprised. (Pause). Now it will be your turn to tell me about different times you felt a certain way. Whatever you tell me will not be repeated to anyone else." A second emotion vignette was provided, if the child did not seem to understand the task. Children were then asked by the experimenter, "Can you tell me a time when you were ________________?" Children were asked to respond to three basic emotion situations (i.e., afraid, happy, sad) and three complex, self-conscious emotions (i.e., embarrassed, guilty, proud).

Children's responses were audio-recorded verbatim and coded by two raters, with inter-rater reliability ranging between .89 to .96 across the DVs. Using a coding scheme adapted from Losh and Capps (2006), each response was coded for appropriateness of the content (0-3), length in number of clauses, causal inferences, and number of prompts needed to elicit a response. Additionally, we examined whether children mentioned an active audience present (e.g., the situation was judged negatively by someone else) and whether they mentioned the violation of a social convention or social norm.

### *Theory of Mind Measure*

The Faux Pas Test-Child Version (Baron-Cohen, O'Riordan, Stone, Jones, & Plaisted, 1999) was used to measure advanced (second-order) ToM. Using this measure, children were asked to listen to 10 short scenarios where one of the characters commits a faux pas. After each scenario, four questions are asked to determine a faux pas detection score. To receive credit towards this score, children had to answer each of the four questions correctly to receive a score of 1 for that scenario. Previous research has shown that the Faux Pas Test has good internal consistency (Cronbach's alpha = 0.91) and test-retest reliability ($r = 0.83$; Soderstrand & Almkvist, 2012).

# RESULTS

## Embarrassment Measures

Preliminary analyses were conducted on the results from the three embarrassment measures in order to confirm the lack of violations of assumptions (e.g., Levene's test for equity of variances, normality of distribution checks). A mixed-model analysis of variance was conducted on the *Audience Awareness* task, with between-subjects variables Diagnostic Group (ASD, NT) and within-subjects variable Type of Audience (Active, Passive, No Audience). Identification of embarrassment in each condition was used as the dependent variable. Results showed a main effect of Type of Audience, $F(2, 90) = 15.69, p < .0001, \eta_p^2 = .27$, and a Type of Audience X Diagnostic Group interaction, $F(2, 90) = 1.92, p < .05, \eta_p^2 = .08$. Follow-up independent-samples t-tests with Bonferroni correction showed that children assigned embarrassment more often to the Active Audience condition than to the other conditions, $t(45) \geq 2.12, p \leq .05$, see Table 4. This provides evidence that all children had an understanding of the role of the audience in the experience of embarrassment. Additionally, children with and without ASD did not differ in their recognition of embarrassment in the Active Audience, $t(45) = -.91, p = .37$, or the No Audience, $t(45) = -.68, p = .49$, conditions. However, children with ASD were more likely than neurotypical children to label vignettes involving a Passive Audience as embarrassing, $t(45) = 2.24, p = .05$. These results are also shown in Table 4.

**Table 4. Children's Responses on the Embarrassment Measure**

| **Audience Awareness Task** | **Mean Proportion Choosing Embarrassment** | | | |
|---|---|---|---|---|
| Condition | ASD | NT | | |
| No Audience | .23 (.43) | .32 (.48) | | |
| Passive Audience | .82 (.39)[b] | .64 (.49)[ab] | | |
| Active Audience | .64 (.49) | .76 (.44) | | |
| **Situational Embarrassment Task** | **Mean Accuracy** | | | |
| Intense Free Response | .69 (.47) | .92 (.27)[a] | | |
| Intense Cues Response | .73 (.45) | .92 (.28)[a] | | |
| Less Intense Free Response | .53 (.50) | .68 (.56) | | |
| Less Intense Cued Response | .52 (.51) | .64 (.49) | | |
| **Recounting Embarrassing Situations Task** | **Means for Coded Variables** | | | |
| Recount Episode | 1 | 2 | 1 | 2 |
| Appropriate Content | 1.4 (1.4) | .78 (1.1) | 2.2 (1.0) | 2.08 (1.4)[a] |
| Number of Causal Inferences | .30 (.47) | .13 (.34) | .36 (.49) | .52 (.48)[ab] |
| Number of Prompts | .73 (.75) | .60 (.98) | .76 (.59) | .60 (.71) |
| Active Audience Mentioned | .09 (.28) | .00 (.00) | .24 (.43) | .16 (.37)[a] |
| Social Convention Mentioned | .17 (.38) | .16 (.37) | .04 (.21) | .12 (.08) |

*Note.* [a] Significant between-subject effect; [b] significant within-subject effect. Appropriate content scores could range from 0 to 3, with 3 reflecting more appropriate content. Causal inferences reflect proportion of recounts that included causal inferences. Number of prompts reflected those given after the initial prompt and ranged from 0 to 3. Standard deviations are in parentheses.

Examining children's other emotional responses to the vignettes (e.g., angry, guilt, happy, sad or neutral) showed that the most used choice besides embarrassment among children with ASD was guilt (36%). In neurotypical children it was also guilt (20%), although some reported sadness (28%). Although children with ASD were more likely than neurotypical children to assign embarrassment to themselves in the Passive Audience condition, children who did not select embarrassment typically reported that the situation would cause them to feel "guilt" regardless of diagnosis.

In the *Situational Embarrassment* task, a mixed-model analysis of variance was conducted, with between-subjects variable Diagnostic Group, and within-subjects variables Type of Response (Free, Forced-Choice) and Intensity (Intense, Less Intense). This analysis revealed a main effect of Diagnostic Group, $F(1, 46) = 4.24, p < .05, \eta_p^2 = .08$, as children with ASD were less accurate than NT children in labeling the embarrassing situations. A main effect of Intensity was also found, $F(1, 46) = 14.46$, $p < .0001, \eta_p^2 = .24$. All children were better at labeling the intense examples of embarrassment than the less intense examples. These results are shown in Table 4. Note that children with and without ASD did not differ in their intensity or duration ratings of the situations, $t(45) \leq -.91$, $p \geq .37$.

In the *Recounting Embarrassing Situations* task the dependent variables included appropriateness of the content (0-3), number of causal inferences, and number of prompts needed to elicit a response. Additional DVs of interest included whether the children mentioned an active audience present and the violation of a social convention or social norm. All results are shown in Table 4. The between-subjects variable was Diagnostic Group (ASD, NT) and the within-subjects variable was the Episode (i.e., Recount 1, Recount 2) in each analysis of a DV.

In terms of appropriateness of content, a main effect of Episode was found, $F(1, 46) = 5.40, p < .03, \eta_p^2 = .11$, as children gave more appropriate content for their first recount. A main effect of Diagnostic Group was also revealed, $F(1, 46) = 10.89, p < .003, \eta_p^2 = .19$, as children with ASD provided less appropriate content than neurotypical children (see Table 4). In terms of number of causal inferences in their recounts, a main effect of Diagnostic Group was found, $F(1, 46) = 4.47, p < .04, \eta_p^2 = .09$, as was a Diagnostic Group X Recount Episode interaction, $F(1, 46) = 4.19, p < .05, \eta_p^2 = .08$. Overall, children with ASD provided recounts with fewer causal inferences, and were especially limited in their second recount episode (see Table 4).

Additional analyses showed no significant difference between the children in terms of number of prompts needed beyond the initial prompt to recount an episode, nor were there significant differences in whether children mentioned a violation of social convention in their recounting of an embarrassing episode. In general, children did not need additional prompts beyond the initial one to elicit the recount, and children typically did not mention a violation of a social convention in an explicit way. However, there was a significant main effect of Diagnostic Group in terms of whether they mentioned an active audience in their recounts, $F(1, 46) = 3.91, p = .05, \eta_p^2 = .08$. Children with ASD were less likely to mention it in their recounts than NT children.

## Relations between Individual Characteristics Embarrassment Task Performance

Across the embarrassment measure, the only significant relations found were for children with ASD. Results showed that the ability to label the Active Audience condition correctly in the *Audience Awareness* task was negatively related to higher SRS-2 T-scores, $r(21) = -0.53, p < .01$, and positively related to faux pas (ToM) detection, $r(21) = 0.47, p < .02$. Thus, greater ASD symptomatology as measured by the SRS-2 was found to be associated with less ability to accurately label embarrassing situations in the active audience condition. Greater ToM ability was associated with better ability to choose embarrassment as the emotion the participant would imagine experiencing when exposed to an embarrassing act with an active audience (i.e., judged the act negatively) present. No other significant relations were found between performance on these two tasks and FSIQ, age, other ASD symptomatology measures, and ToM scores. No significant relations were found between these scores and neurotypical children's performance across the embarrassment measure.

## DISCUSSION

The purpose of this study was to isolate the emotional components of embarrassment in order to examine the differences in understanding and recounting the emotion in children with and without ASD. Specifically, this study examined whether children with ASD and neurotypical children were aware of the role of the audience when asked to imagine themselves in embarrassing situations, whether children were able to distinguish between intense and mildly embarrassing situations happening to another child, and the extent to which children could recount their own embarrassing experiences. Additionally, this study examined the relations between ASD symptomatology, ToM, and other individual factors (FSIQ, age) on children's responses across the embarrassment tasks.

The findings from the *Audience Awareness* task revealed that both children with and without ASD understood an active (derisive) audience's impact on the experience of embarrassment. Indeed, all children found the active audience vignette the most embarrassing, indicating that both children with ASD and neurotypical children had a basic understanding of a judgmental audience's impact on the experience of embarrassment. When no audience was present, children with ASD did not differ from neurotypical children in their assignment of embarrassment to the situation, suggesting that they understood that without an audience present they would have been less likely to experience embarrassment. These findings support past research (e.g., Hillier & Allinson, 2002b) by demonstrating that children with ASD are able to sufficiently understand some facets of the complex emotion of embarrassment.

However, children with ASD differed significantly from neurotypical children in that they were more likely to find the passive audience vignette embarrassing. This finding is consistent with Hillier and Allinson's (2002a) results to the extent that they found that children with ASD were more likely than neurotypical children to report non-embarrassing scenarios as embarrassing. The increased likelihood of finding the passive audience vignette embarrassing in children with ASD is consistent with the growing trend in the current literature that suggests high functioning children with

ASD may be more sensitive and susceptible to feelings of embarrassment (or other complex emotions, Davidson et al., 2018), although it is not clear if this is due to a lack of understanding about the nuances of embarrassment.

The *Situational Embarrassment* task also revealed similarities and differences between children with ASD and neurotypical children. Consistent with previous research, children with ASD were less able to identify embarrassing situations than neurotypical children (Hillier & Allinson, 2002a). However, when children did label a situation embarrassing, neurotypical children and children with ASD did not differ in their ratings of the intensity or duration of the emotion (i.e., the degree to which the protagonist felt embarrassment in the situation and how long the feeling would last). These results provide evidence that all children understood how intensity of the embarrassing situation (i.e., situations that should produce more or less embarrassment) affects one's perception of it. Furthermore, all children were better at labeling (i.e., attributing embarrassment) in more intensely embarrassing situations than more mildly embarrassing situations. Nevertheless, children with ASD were less accurate in identifying embarrassing situations overall.

Additional findings were revealed in the *Recounting Embarrassing Situations* task. Children with ASD struggled the most with this task. When asked to recount two personal experiences of feeling embarrassed, children with ASD provided less appropriate content than children without ASD. Also noteworthy, children with ASD provided recounts with significantly fewer causal inferences and were especially limited in their second recount. These findings are consistent with past research that found that children with ASD struggled the most with justifying why particular scenarios or experiences were embarrassing (Hillier & Allinson, 2002a; Losh & Capps, 2006).

It is important to understand why children with ASD may have experienced the most difficulty when asked to recount their own experiences of embarrassment. When it is presented to them in a form of a scenario, especially one with an active (derisive) audience present, children can use the context as an explicit means for recognizing embarrassment. However, without those explicit cues they may not recognize the need to use them or report them in their recounts. Thus, our results indicate that children's understanding of embarrassment is best examined using a variety of measures as performance on one task may not match up to their performance on another.

In terms of the mechanisms that underlie children's understanding of embarrassment, we examined the much-touted association between ToM and embarrassment. Thus, we made a concerted effort to assess ToM ability in children, along with other individual characteristics (ASD symptomatology, FSIQ, age) in relation to their responses on the embarrassment tasks. Overall, we found that greater ToM ability was associated with accurately choosing embarrassment as the emotion the child would imagine experiencing when exposed to an embarrassing act with an active audience present. This finding confirms and expands past research by demonstrating, rather that hypothesizing, that better developed ToM skills enables children to have a more accurate and complex understanding of the role of an active (derisive) audience in embarrassing situations. Furthermore, the current study demonstrated that greater ASD symptomatology was associated with less ability to accurately label embarrassing situations in the active audience condition. However, the general lack of relations between the individual characteristics we examined and children's understanding of embarrassment suggest that future research may want to examine the role other factors play. For example, it would be valuable to determine why children with ASD found the passive audience situation more embarrassing than neurotypical children. Was this due to an over-sensitivity to embarrassment or to other factors (e.g., lack of understanding about the role of the audience)?

## Limitations and Future Directions

Although we believe our results are compelling, a few limitations should be noted. One potential issue was the small sample size, although the size of our participant pool was within the range of other studies researching emotion processing in children with ASD. Additionally, it will be important for future research to examine the role linguistic factors may play on tasks assessing children's understanding of embarrassment. Although our measure of FSIQ included a measure of receptive language proficiency that all children scored within their age range on, it is possible that other language factors play a role in children's ability to understand situational contexts and to communicate about embarrassing situations in their own lives. Finally, all of our children with ASD were high functioning. Much less is known about how lower-functioning children with ASD understand and process complex emotions such as embarrassment.

Additional suggestions for future research include studying the relations between how children with ASD process and respond to embarrassing situations across artificial (lab) and real-life scenarios, paying particular attention to children's conception of the importance of an audience (active or passive) across experiences. Similarly, future studies should continue to explore the possibility that children with ASD experience embarrassment to a broader array of events (e.g., with a passive audience present) and what, if anything, this means for children with ASD in terms of their experiences with other complex, self-conscious (e.g., guilt, shame) emotions.

## Conclusion and Implications

The present study was able to expand upon previous findings by directly analyzing children's ability to identify and comprehend embarrassment in multiple conditions. Embarrassment is an important emotional experience that guides our ability to navigate complex social environments. If those with ASD struggle to comprehend embarrassment, then this can impact their ability to operate within social settings. With a better understanding of the way children with ASD experience embarrassment and other complex emotions, interventions could specifically target facets that those with ASD commonly struggle with. Our results found that children with ASD are able to understand the impact of an active audience in embarrassing vignettes but may differ from other children in their views about the presence of a passive audience in embarrassing situations. Additional differences were found in children's recounting of embarrassing situations. Although more research is needed, the results of this study offer a new view into how children with ASD process and store complex emotional information, how well they understand and label a complex emotion, and how well they understand this emotion in others.

## REFERENCES

American Psychiatric Association. 2000. *Diagnostic and Statistical Manual of Mental Disorders.* Arlington: American Psychiatric Association.

American Psychiatric Association. 2013. *Diagnostic and Statistical Manual of Mental Disorders.* Arlington: American Psychiatric Association.

Baron-Cohen, Simon, Michelle O'Riordan, Valerie Stone, Rosie Jones, and Kate Plaisted. 1999. "Recognition of Faux Pas by Normally Developing Children and Children with Asperger Syndrome or High-Functioning Autism" *Journal of Autism and Developmental Disorders* 29:407-18. doi:10.1023/a:1023035012436.

Beeger, Sander, Carolien Rieffe, Mark Meerum, and Lex Stockmann. 2006. "Attention to Facial Emotion Expressions in Children with Autism". *Autism* 10:37-51. doi:10.1177/1362361306057862.

Bennett, Mark. 1989. "Children's Self-attribution of Embarrassment." *British Journal of Developmental Psychology* 7:207-17. https://loyola-primo.hosted.exlibrisgroup.com/permalink/f/16h7vb8/TN_wj10.1111/j.2044-835X.1989.tb00801.x.

Bennett, Mark and Karen Gillingham. 1991. "The Role of Self-Focused Attention in Children's Attribution of Social Emotions to the Self." *The Journal of Genetic Psychology* 152:303-09. doi:10.1080/00221325.1991.9914688.

Bennett, Mark, Nicola Yuill, Robin Banerjee, and Susan Thomson. 1998. "Children's Understanding of Extended Identity." *Developmental Psychology* 34:322-31. doi:10.1037/0012-1649.34.2.322.

Capps, Lisa, Nurit Yirmiya, and Marian Sigman. 1992. "Understanding of Simple and Complex Emotions in Non-Retarded Children with

Autism." *Child Psychology & Psychiatry & Allied Disciplines* 33:1169–82. doi:10.1111/j.1469-7610.1992.tb00936.x.

Chandler, Susie, Tony Charman, Gillian Baird, Emily Simonoff, Tom Loucas, David Meldrum, Mimi Scott, and Andrew Pickles. 2007. "Validation of the Social Communication Questionnaire in a Population Cohort of Children with Autism Spectrum Disorders." *Journal of the American Academy of Child & Adolescent Psychiatry* 115:1324-32. doi: 10.1177/0963721412454874.

Colonnesi, Cristina, Iris M Engelhard, and Susan M Bögels. 2010. "Development in Children's Attribution of Embarrassment and the Relationship with Theory of Mind and Shyness." *Cognition and Emotion* 24:514-21. doi:10.1080/02699930902847151.

Constantino, John M. and Christian P. Gruber. 2012. *Social Responsiveness Scale-Second Edition (SRS-2)*. Torrance, CA: Western Psychological Services.

Davidson, Denise. 2006. "The Role of Basic, Self-Conscious and Self-Conscious Evaluative Emotions in Children's Memory an Understanding of Emotion. *Motivation and Emotion* 30:237-47. doi:10.1007/s11031-006-9037-6.

Davidson, Denise, Elizabeth Hilvert, Ieva Misiunaite, and Michael Giordano. 2018. "Proneness to guilt, shame, and pride in children with Autism Spectrum Disorders and neurotypical children." *Autism Research* 11:883-92. doi:10.1002/aur.1937.

Feinberg, Matthew M., Robb Willer, and Dacher Keltner. 2011. "Flustered and Faithful: Embarrassment as a Signal of Prosociality." *Journal of Personality and Social Psychology* 102:81-97. doi:10.1037/a0025403.

Gilovich, Thomas, and Kenneth Savitsky. 2000. "The Spotlight Effect in Social Judgment: An Egocentric Bias in Estimates of the Salience of One's Own Actions and Appearance." *Journal of Personality and Social Psychology* 78:211-22. doi:10.1037/0022-3514.78.2.211.

Goffman, Erving. (1956). "Embarrassment and Social Organization." *American Journal of Sociology* 62:264-71. doi:10.1086/222003.

Hillier, Ashleigh and Lesley Allinson. 2002a. "Understanding Embarrassment Among Those with Autism: Breaking Down the

Complex Emotion of Embarrassment Among Those with Autism." *Journal of Autism and Development Disorders* 32:583-92. http://flagship.luc.edu/login?url=https://search.ebscohost.com/login.aspx?direct=true&db=rzh&AN=106080157&site=ehost-live.

Hillier, Ashleigh and Lesley Allinson. 2002b. "Beyond Expectations: Autism, Understanding Embarrassment, and the Relationship with Theory of Mind." *Autism* 6:299-13. doi:10.1177/1362361302006003007.

Keltner, Dacher and Brenda Buswell. 1997. "Embarrassment: Its Distinct Form and Appeasement Function." *Psychological Bulletin* 122:250-70. doi:10.1037/0033-2909.122.3.250.

Lagattuta, Kristen H. and Ross A. Thomson. 2007. "The Development of Self-Conscious Emotions: Cognitive Processes and Social Influences." In *The Self-Conscious Emotions: Theory and Research,* 91-113. New York: Guilford Press.

Lewis, Michael. 2008. "Self-conscious emotions: Embarrassment, pride, shame, and guilt. In *Handbook of emotions*, 742-56. New York: Guilford Press.

Lord, Catherine and Christina Corsello. 2005. "Diagnostic instruments in Autistic Spectrum Disorders." *Handbook of Autism and pervasive developmental disorders*, 730-71. New York: Wiley.

Losh, Molly and Lisa Capps. 2006. "Understanding of Emotional Experience in Autism: Insights from the Personal Accounts of High-functioning Children with Autism." *Developmental Psychology* 43:809-18. doi:10.1037/0012-1649.42.5.809.

Miller, Rowland S. 1996. *Embarrassment: Poise and Peril in Everyday Life. Emotions and Social Behavoir.* New York: Guilford Press.

Miller, Rowland S. 2007. "Is Embarrassment a Blessing or a Curse?" In *the Self-Conscious Emotions: Theory and Research*, 245-62. New York: Guilford Press.

Nadar-Grosbois, Nathalie and James M. Day. 2011. Emotional Cognition: Theory of mind and Face Recognition. *International handbook of Autism and pervasive developmental disorders* 127-57.

Reddy, Vasudevi. 2000. "Coyness in Early Infancy." *Developmental Science* 3:186-92. doi:10.1111/1467-7687.00112.

Rutter, Michael, Anthony Bailey, and Catherine Lord. 2003. *The Social Communication Questionnaire.* Los Angeles: Western Psychological Services.

Schopler, Eric, Mary E. Van Bourgondien, Glenna J. Wellman, and Steven R. Love. 2010. *Childhood Autism Rating Scale.* Los Angeles: Western Psychological Services.

Soderstand, Peter and Ove Almkvist. 2012. "Psychometric Data on the Eyes Test, Faux Pas Test, and the Dewey Social Stories Test in a population-based Swedish Adult Sample." *Nordic Psychology* 62:30-43. doi:10.1080/19012276.2012.693729.

Speer, Leslie L., Anne E. Cook, William M. McMahon, and Elaine Clark. 2007. "Face Processing in Children with Autism: Effects of Stimulus Contents and Type." *Autism* 11:265-77. doi:10.1177/136236130 7076925.

Tangney, June P. and Rhonda L. Dearing. 2002. *Shame and Guilt.* Emotions and Social Behavior. New York: Guilford Press.

Tell, Dina, Denise Davidson, and Linda A. Camras. 2014. "Recognition of Emotion from Facial Expressions with Direct or Averted Eye Gaze and Varying Expression Intensities in Children with Autism Spectrum Disorder and Typically Developing Children." *Autism Research and Treatment* 2014: 1-11. doi:10.11.55/2014/816137.

Tracy, Jessica L., Richard W. Robins, and June Price. 2007. *The Self-Conscious Emotions: Theory and Research.* New York: Guilford Press.

Wechsler, David. 2011. *Wechsler Abbreviated Scale of Intelligence (WASI-II).* San Antonio: NCS, Pearson.

## BIOGRAPHICAL SKETCH

***Denise Davidson***

**Affiliation:** Loyola University Chicago

**Education:** BS, MS, PhD in Psychology

**Research and Professional Experience:** Please see my professional website: https://davidsonautismlab.weebly.com

**Professional Appointments:** Loyola University Chicago

**Publications from the Last 3 Years:**

Davidson, D., Hilvert, E., Misiunaite, I., & Giordano, M. (2018). Proneness to shame, guilt and pride in children with Autism Spectrum Disorders and neurotypical children, *Autism Research,* 11, 883-892. doi: 10.1002/aur.1937 [Peer Reviewed].

Davidson, D., Hilvert, E., Misunaite, I., Kerby, K., & Giordano, M. (2019). Recognition of facial emotions on human and canine faces in children with and without Autism Spectrum Disorders. *Motivation and Emotion,* 43, 191-202. doi: https://doi.org/10.1007/s11031-018-9736-9 [Peer reviewed].

Davidson, D., Hughes, K. S., Misiunaite, I., Hilvert, E., & Shuldiner, A. (2018). Body image and life satisfaction in Amish, Catholic, and Non-religious Women. *Journal of Amish and Anabaptist Studies,* 6, 174-191. doi: https://kb.osu.edu/handle/1811/8709 [Peer reviewed].

Davidson, D., Rainey, V., Vanegas, S. B., & Hilvert, E. (2017). The effects of type of instructions, animacy cues, and dimensionality of objects on the shape bias in children. *Infant and Child Development.* https://doi.1002/icd.2044 [Peer Reviewed].

Davidson, D., Vanegas, S. B., & Hilvert, E. (2017). Proneness to self-conscious emotions in adults with and without Autism traits. *Journal of Autism and Developmental Disorders,* 47, 3392-3404. doi:10.1007/s10803-017-3260-8 [Peer Reviewed].

Davidson, D., Vanegas, S. B., Hilvert, E. & Misiunaite, I. (2017). "I read the book last week." The role of dominant language and receptive vocabulary on morphosyntactic awareness in monolingual and bilingual children. *Bilingualism: Language and Cognition,* 20, 1045-1062. doi:10.1017/S136672891600078X [Peer Reviewed].

Davidson, D., Vanegas, S. B., Hilvert, E., Rainey, V. R., & Misiunaite, I. (2019). Examination of monolingual (English) and bilingual (English/Spanish; English/Urdu) children's syntactic awareness. *Journal of Child Language,* 46, 682-706. doi: 10.1017/S03050 00919000059 [Peer reviewed].

Hilvert, E., Davidson, D., & Gámez, P. B. (2016). Examination of script and non-script based narrative retellings in children with Autism Spectrum Disorders. *Research in Autism Spectrum Disorders.* 30, 79-92. doi:10.1016/j.rasd.2016.06.002 [Peer Reviewed].

Hilvert, E., Davidson, D., & Scott, C. M. (2019). An in-depth analysis of expository writing in children with and without Autism Spectrum Disorders. *Journal of Autism and Developmental Disorders,* 49, 3412-3425. doi: https://doi.org/10.1007/s10803-019-04057-2 [Peer Reviewed].

Hilvert, E., Davidson, D., Scott, C. M., & Gamez, P. (2019). Assessment of personal narrative writing in children with and without Autism Spectrum Disorder. *Research on Autism Spectrum Disorders,* 69, https://doi.org/10.1016/j.rasd.2019.101453 [Peer reviewed].

In: Understanding Children with Autism … ISBN: 978-1-53617-647-6
Editor: Anne Bourque 

*Chapter 7*

# Diet–Related Issues with Autism Spectrum Disorder

***Seema Siddiqi and Asna Urooj****
Department of Studies in Food Science and Nutrition,
University of Mysore, Mysore, Karnataka, India

## Abstract

Autism Spectrum Disorder (ASD) is the fastest growing developmental disability that affects children particularly prior to the age of three in the areas of verbal & non-verbal communication, social interactions, physical abnormalities, sensory impairments & cognitive function. Along with these issues, dietary risk factors also affect the normal development of the children which make them vulnerable to serious nutritional deficiencies. Diet related issues like gastro-intestinal complications, leaky-guts; micro-biota composition, food neo-phobia, selective or picky eating habits and certain foods (gluten, casein) could aggravate with the symptoms of ASD and could be developed into a major and recurrent concern as reported by the parents or caretakers of ASD. Despite recent advances in the diagnostic tools & knowledge of pivotal factors, the exact etiology of autism remains unidentified, but it is predicted

* Corresponding Author's E-mail: asnau321@gmail.com.

to be due to exposure to genetic susceptibility, medical co-morbidities & other environmental factors. Presently there is no known therapy to treat ASD, however children with this disorder do progress & the diverse symptoms related to it can be improved with primary intervention & treatments. Professionals researching on ASD have clearly indicated that early diagnosis & intervention programs including the pharmacological & non-conventional methods viz; occupational, pragmatic skills along with dietary modifications may lead to significant improvement outcomes & better levels of functioning for children with ASD, as they reach their adulthood. Dietary related risk factors & how food plays a pivotal role in reducing the symptoms of ASD is the new emerging area of research work which has to be substantially validated through evidence based diets. With respect to dietary issues, awareness on eating habits and feeding problems experienced by ASD children need to be emphasized among parents or guardians of children as the road to recovery in every ailment is through diet.

**Keywords:** feeding behavior, dietary risk factors, elimination diets, dietary supplements

## INTRODUCTION

Autism is one of five developmental disorders included under the umbrella of the Pervasive Developmental Disorders (PDDs). In addition to ASD, other disorders in this family are Asperger's Syndrome, Rett's Disorder, and Childhood Disintegrative Disorder. These conditions lead on to disabilities in virtually all the psychological and behavioral sectors with protuberant disturbances in social, communicative and cognitive ranges. Autism spectrum disorders are neuro-developmental disorders characterized by series of impairments in socialization, communication and repetitive behavior (APA, DSM, 2013). Historically, ASD was considered a "mysterious" brain disorder, entailing that it begins and ends in the brain. Though autism had existed much early, it was only described & named in the 1950's as evident by its special & specific characteristics. The word 'autism' was first used by Bleuler, a Swiss psychiatrist in 1911 to refer to schizophrenia. The historical perspective of ASD in India was first described by Leo Kanner in 1943 in his classic report of 11 children with "autistic disturbances of affective contact." Another pediatrician Ronald observed similar characteristics of autistic children in Darjeeling to that made by Kanner & made a fact that the difficulties experienced by autistic children can have an overall lifelong impact on their mental personality (Purkayastha & Girimaji et al., 1997).

Center for Autism, India (Action for Autism) the current statistics (2010 data) on prevalence of autism & its spectrum disorders is 1 out of 80 children. According to (Autism Society of America), it is four times more prevalent in boys than girls in the United States. Incidence extrapolations for India for Autism: 11,914 per year, 250 per month, 57 per week, 8 per day, 1.4 per hour. Autism is more common than Down syndrome, which occurs in 1 out of 800 births. Estimates of 15 per 10,000 are now typical rising to 64 per 10,000 or even higher if the entire spectrum is included. This steep rise in the occurrence of the disorder could be attributed to the diagnostic tools & treatment strategies employed to correct the conditions (ADDM & CDC, 2012).

## DIAGNOSIS

Autism can be diagnosed in infants as young as 1 year old by observation using proper questionnaires & screening tools. A developmental pediatrician, psychologist, neurologist or psychiatrist familiar with developmental disorders can make a diagnosis. At first glance, some ASD children may appear to have an intellectual frailty, sensory processing issues, or problems with hearing or vision; therefore, it is very important to differentiate ASD from other disorders, as suitable treatment programs (interventions) can be provided based on the accuracy and early diagnosis (Srinath & Choudhary et al., 1989). ASD cannot be managed by single therapist; it requires multi-dimensional approach of various disciplines to focus on the issues and to bring about positive outcomes. Therefore, the management team for ASD is as shown in the Figure 1.

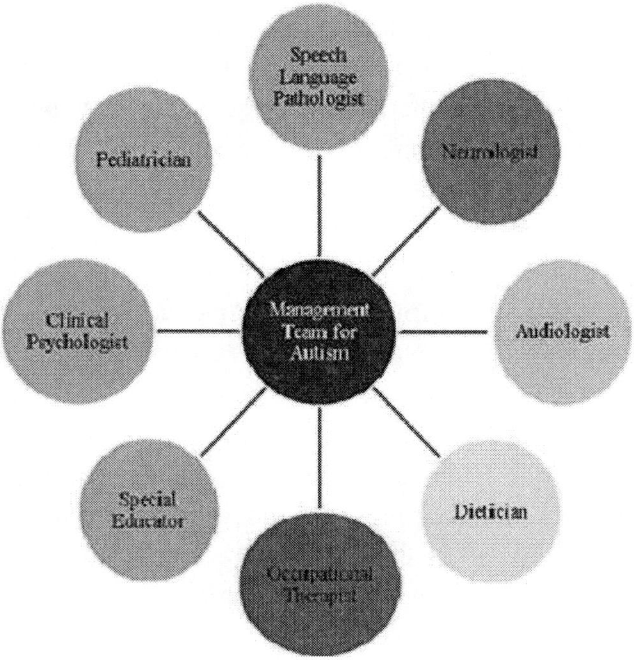


Figure 1: Management Team for Autism.

There is no medical test existing to diagnose ASD because many of the behaviors allied with autism are common to other disorders, therefore an accurate diagnosis must be based on observation of the individual's communication, social interaction, and his or her activities and interests. Wide ranges of screening and diagnostic instrument for diagnosis of ASD have been devised during the last decades. It is also observed that clinical based screening is the most common reported method to diagnose ASD (Howlin & Moorre, 1997). In India, in the recent years, Indian Scale for Assessment of Autism (ISSA) was developed at NIMH (National Institute for Mental Health, Secunderabad). It is a standardized tool with high degree of reliability and validity for issuance of disability certificate for persons with autism in India (Russell & Daniel et al., 2010).

However, an initial medical assessment typically includes; a medical history of the mother's pregnancy, developmental milestones, eating and sleeping habits, co-ordination issues, stomach and bowel functioning, sensory challenges, allergies, medical illnesses, including ear infections and seizures, any family history of developmental disorders, etc.

## CAUSATIVE FACTORS

Despite recent advances in the diagnostic tools & knowledge of pivotal factors, the exact etiology of ASD remains unidentified, but it is assumed to be due to exposure to genetic susceptibility, medical co-morbidities & other environmental factors. Researchers claim that there is no known single cause for autism spectrum disorder, but it is generally accepted that it is caused by abnormalities in brain structure or function. However, there is every reason to hope in the coming time to know the exact cause of ASD, which in turn will lead to more effective treatments, appropriate services & improvements in the lives of those affected by autism. Autism spectrum disorder impacts the nervous system and affects the overall social, cognitive, emotional, and physical health of the affected individual. The range and severity of symptoms can vary widely among individuals. Common symptoms include difficulty with communication & social interactions, obsessive interests and repetitive stereotyped behaviors along with various co-occurring physical and nutritional related conditions (Siegel, 1997).

## GENERAL NUTRITIONAL STATUS

Numerous research papers discussing the dietary status of children affected with ASD have contradictory results on the nutritional status and have reported that though the adequacy/deficiency of macronutrients does not vary much among the typically developing and ASD children; but in terms of micronutrients, there are significant differences. A classical longitudinal study by (Massaroa and Raiten, 1986) reported higher intake of carbohydrates, proteins and total energy requirements and lower levels of fats. However, the nutritional status of ASD children and typically developing children had similar overall nutrient adequacies. Another study by (Morales et al., 2014) compared the nutrient intakes and body mass index (BMI) of Autism Spectrum Disorder (ASD) children and typically developing (TD) children. This was a case control study which was studied among (n=40) ASD children and (n=113) TD children in the age group of 6-10 years. The study evaluated the nutrient intakes of the two groups and found that there were significant differences between the vital nutrients. The results of the study projected lower intakes of fluoride and vitamin E levels. The study also assessed the overall quality of diet and its impact on dietary restriction. Many other studies have also reported similar conclusions about the nutritional profile of the children with ASD (Zimmer et al., 2012; Levy et al., 2007 Emond et al., 2010 & Schmitt et al., 2008). All the findings of these studies suggest that despite food selectivity and repetitive behavior which is a characteristic feature of ASD children, the energy and macronutrient requirements are well fulfilled. However, other authors have reported the extent of inadequate intake of micronutrients-Folic acid, Niacin, Iron, B6, Riboflavin (Herndon et al., 2009; Wei et al., 2010; Shearer et al., 1982 & Cornish et al., 1998) among these children. Bandini et al., 2010; Ho et al., 1997; Johnson et al., 2008; Lindsay et al., 2006 have reported lower intake of Calcium, Vitamin A, C and D levels.

## Dietary Problems in ASD

In addition to the socio-behavioral problems, diet-related issues are also a recurrent concern as reported by the parents or caretakers of ASD populations (Bandini et al., 2010; Ledford and Gast 2006). Physical conditions observed in individuals with ASD include diarrhea, constipation, bloating, GI discomfort, leaky-gut; recurrent infections, sleeping pattern alterations, and generalized inflammation/pain. Along with these, ASD children are also affected by micronutrient deficiencies, feeding problems, food neo-phobia, increased sensory problems, persistence to food presentations, selective or picky eating habits and decreased food varieties (Feingold & Song et al., 2002). All these dietary risk factors affect the normal development of the children which make them vulnerable to serious nutritional deficiencies. The sequence of nutritional related complications is as shown in the Figure 2. Therefore, categorizing ASD as a whole body disorder comprehends what happens inside the body and cells & how it affects the brain and how the food fed to a child affects the body and its biochemistry is the need of the hour for proposing the nutritional intervention studies.

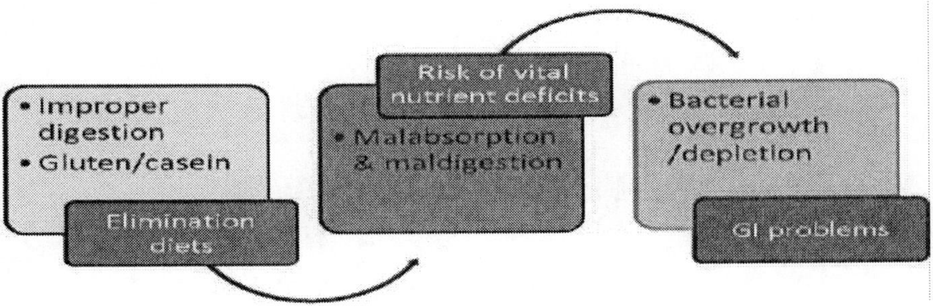


Figure 2: Sequence of Nutritional related problems in Autism.

## How Food Matters

Food has direct contact with and also immediately affects the gut. Good health is synonymous with a healthy diet and indeed good digestion is critical. Many studies reports that impaired digestion and GI health are associated with advancing physiological and behavioral symptoms among ASD children. Leaky-gut, mal-absorption of nutrients, inflammatory responses to foods that are not broken down, and thus resulting in burdening the detoxification system are all associated with poor digestion. Nutrients are crucial to all biochemical and brain function. Therefore, optimal nutritional status requires the consumption of nutrient dense food and proper digestion to breakdown and absorbs those foods. Poor digestion often results from environmental factors which include genetic susceptibility, absence of beneficial bacteria, inflammation, and immune system response to certain foods, and studies have shown leaky-gut, low levels of beneficial flora, inflammation and immune response to food in children with ASD. Additionally, the response to certain foods such as gluten and casein can create an opiate or inflammatory reaction that can affect the brain. Various physiological parameters observed in ASD include auto-immune reactions, food reactions, diagnostic connection of upper GI disease, abnormal stools, autistic entero-colitis, leaky-gut syndrome, excessive inflammation, aberrant glutathione levels, irregular metal, mineral levels, etc. (Jepson and Johnson, 2007) all supporting the importance of the gut micro-biome. The afore mentioned parameters are either influenced by micro-biota or vice versa, revealing the tantalizing link between ASD and gut micro-biome.

## FEEDING PROBLEMS

Feeding problems frequently occur in childhood, studies report around 25–35% of typically developing children experiences feeding issues and up to 80% of those with developmental delay. An unusual complex interactional model with biological vulnerabilities occurs in ASD due to dysfunction in cognitive, sensory and emotional response interacting with dysfunctional attachment and learnt behaviors and this is the basal cause of feeding problems in ASD. Children with ASD have problems of food selectivity, food refusal, behavioral meal problems and restricted dietary intake implying risk of nutritional deficiencies disorders. Sarah Hurwitz (1998) describes feeding problems in children with ASD from milder to severe forms which can have negative impact on their nutritional status. The common issues of feeding as experienced by parents includes swallowing difficulties, vomiting, food neo-phobia, emotional under-eating or over-eating which makes them difficult to manage their children (Soumyanath,2014).Along with this; Pica, anorectic behavior, complete food refusal as well as unusual food restriction and preferences are also common feeding issues in ASD children. Effective treatment therefore requires a novel multifaceted approach that can address each of these areas.

# DIETARY - RISK FACTORS

The dietary offending risk factors which aggravate the physical conditions in ASD patients include microbial overgrowth, opiates, food additives, phenolic foods, salicylates, oxalates, amines & glutamines. In addition to these, there are certain food substances (most notably gluten and casein) which are known to trigger the problems in ASD, and should therefore be eliminated in the diets.

Multiple studies have reported GI abnormalities in the gut of ASD children compared with healthy or sibling controls. A study by Valenci-McDermott et al., 2006 and Adams et al., 2004;have indicated that 70% of children with ASD having a history of GI complaints, against 28% of neuro-typical controls, and that GI symptoms are strongly correlated with the severity of ASD (r 0·59; P<0·001). The GI abnormalities found in ASD children include mal-absorption, mal-digestion, microbial overgrowth (fungal, bacterial and viral) and abnormal intestinal permeability. These events could cause symptoms including diarrhea, constipation, gas and belching, probing and visibly undigested foods. Microbial overgrowth includes bacteria, fungi & yeast which can cause gut inflammation & is also associated with decreased gut function. Many studies have indicated that overgrowth of yeast is common in ASD children as it is triggered due to overuse of antibiotics. Toxins of yeast can cross the blood brain barrier & can cause symptoms ranging from drunken behaviors to affecting energy levels & critical thinking. The GI complications associated with them are mal-absorption, mal-digestion and leaky-gut syndrome. The events of symptoms include diarrhea, constipation, bloating, gastric irritability, feeding problems, esophageal reflux (Adam & Powell et al., 2011). Several metabolic abnormalities have been found in ASD children, which include defects in methylation, disturbed concentration of amino acids in plasma and oxidative stress. Abnormal sulfur metabolism, lower concentrations of mammalian – microbial co-metabolites and a more disturbed concentration of amino acids in plasma, active nicotinic acid metabolism, have also been found in ASD individuals.

Another important dietary risk factor includes food allergy, where the food antigen leads to a response by T cells and subsequently to an initiation of a food-mediated immune response. A significantly greater incidence of food allergy in ASD patients compared with healthy controls has been reported by ASD parents. A study by Lucarelli et al., (1995) reported that an oral challenge with cows' milk protein results in worsening of some of the behavioral symptoms of ASD children, and that these children express significantly higher serum levels of IgA, IgG and IgM for casein and IgA for lactalbumin and b-lactoglobulin compared with typically developing children. Development of lesions in the ileum that consist of enlarged lymphoid nodules containing large collections of lymphocytes in the GI lymphoid tissues adjacent to Peyer's patches has been associated with food allergy as reported by Sabra et al., (2012). According to this study food allergy is the critical contributing factor for these above mentioned conditions. These GI lesions would allow the entry of food antigens across the inflamed mucosa of the bowel and elicit an inflammatory response in the GI tract.

There are certain protein component when ingested can bring about various digestive problems, such as gluten, casein. The main sources of these are wheat, rye, barley, commercial oats and dairy products. In people who are compromised for the indigestion of these proteins including the ASD ones, consumption of these proteins can cause inflammation of the gastrointestinal lining & other associated complications of the gut like pain, diarrhea, bloating, etc. These problems are emerged due to the formation of opiates which are the results of protein indigestion. Opiates or morphine like compounds can initiate irritability, foggy thinking & inattentiveness in ASD children.

## Role of Food in Alleviating the Symptoms

Though there are no effective medications or treatments to cure or relieve the core symptoms of ASD, other alternative treatments like occupational therapies, sensory integration therapies, pragmatic skill therapies to facilitate language & increase social interactions, dietary intervention through supplementation or elimination of certain diets can be used to improve the conditions of ASD. It has been noted, 'wherethere is no cure, there are hundred treatments'. Thus many studies have been postulated with theories & hypothesized on the dietary aspects & its relationship on overcoming the episodes of ASD symptoms.

The road to recovery begins with proper diet not only in medical related diseased conditions but also controls well in ASD cases too. In this present context, autistic individuals are subjected to various alternative therapies with a prime focus on dietary approaches. The physical conditions can be aggravated among individuals with ASD with digestive problems, imbalanced biochemistry within the body and nutritional deficiencies. Therefore, altering food choices & possible food interventions could help in improving the symptoms both physical and as well as behavioral.

A healthy diet is essential for optimal health & to accomplish this proper digestion is critical. The physiological and behavioral symptoms of ASD in many cases may start from impaired digestion and GI ill health. Food has direct contact & immediately affects the gut, which is an essential component to understand and address in ASD. The gut breaks down the food so that the nutrients are made available to the body which is needed to support biochemical processes and allow the brain to function properly. The largest part of the immune system is found in the gut; a system often imbalanced in ASD causing an inability to fight against viruses, yeast, and other pathogens properly while contributing an overactive inflammatory and allergic response. Foods which are not properly digested in the body can create inflammation & the contaminants in the gut from bad bacteria and yeast can produce off toxins that affect the brain. About 90% of serotonin (calming brain chemical/hormone) is found in the gut, which is essential in maintaining normal activity of the brain & is lacking in ASD patients. Poor digestion can lead to various manifestations such as leaky-gut, mal-absorption of nutrients, lack/low levels of beneficial bacteria, inflammatory responses to foods that are not broken down, and a burden to the detoxification system.

## Dietary Treatments

As ASD patients are currently subjected to numerous 'alternative interventions' by caregivers and researchers, many are specifically aim at diet & are intended in improving the gut health. According to a study by Wheeler et al.,(2006) treating the digestive system abnormalities has tremendously decreased the core symptoms of autism & other spectrum disorders. In this present context, the described interventions include gluten-free and casein-free diets, dietary supplementation with essential fatty acids, pre and probiotics, vitamins & minerals.

## Elimination Diets

While nutritional therapies & dietary restrictions may not completely cure the symptoms, they can definitely be beneficial as complementary to other treatments. Elimination diets are based primarily on reducing or completely removing the foods from the diet that triggers the symptoms, mostly those ones causing food intolerance or allergies. GFCF (gluten free & casein free) foods are planned for the ASD cases as the basic elimination diets. A study by Hediger et al.(2008) has indicated that the physical conditions are drastically reduced while on GFCF diets in ASD and is considered as the golden diet for these targeted populations.

In addition, there are several other elimination diets which are based on reducing or completely removing those foods from the diet that adversely affect the ASD people. They include Feingold diets whose principle is based on the removal of dyes or food colors, intentional additives, chemical preservatives from the daily diets (Feingold B.F., 1975). Another study by (Elder et al., 2008) indicated a high-fat, low-protein & low-carbohydrate diet called Ketogenic diet used to treat refractory epilepsy which provides 90% of the energy from fats & remaining from proteins & carbohydrates. However, this classical diet should be used under expertise medical & dietician supervision on the patients whose serum ketone bodies level is in controlled limits if not, they can be subjected to risk their lives with a number of metabolic disorders.

(Gottschall, 2004) first introduced specific carbohydrate diet to treat autistic individuals aimed at relieving the symptoms of mal-absorption & preventing the growth of intestinal micro flora. This diet is recommended to restore back the normal functioning of the gut by including only monosaccharide such as fruits, honey, certain vegetables & avoiding complex carbohydrates as they take longer time to get digested. Thus the residual growth may account for microbial overgrowth resulting in excessive production of intestinal mucus secretion thereby causing intestinal dysbiosis & leaky-gut formation (Song Y et al., 2002).

Though ASD is a genetic disorder, certain metabolic disorders aggravates the clinical symptoms & may pose one of the reasons for pathogenesis of ASD such as high concentration of oxalates in the blood serum levels. Oxalates are known to hamper the neurological development & therefore must be limited in ASD (Levy et al., 2007). Low oxalate diets ranging from 40-50mg/day is generally recommended to autistic patients against 250mg/day which is the acceptable daily intake (Barr & Murphy et al., 2002).

## Dietary Supplementations

Mental disorders can begin from various commotions in the body ranging from biochemical reactions, genetic issues to dietary issues, micronutrient deficiencies or nutritional complications (Pauling, 1968). Appropriate supplements therefore, can be recommended to the ASD individuals to ameliorate the symptoms & correct the deficiencies. A study by (Matson et al., 2009) indicates that ASD children consume lesser foods than compare to control counterparts. Due to their selective eating habits & stereotyped behavior problems they are more prone to nutritional deficiency disorders. Hence, there is escalating evidence based research carried out in various foods that can be supplemented to this kind of individuals to prevent nutritional related deficiencies.(Geis et al., 2011) conducted a randomized, double blind, placebo-controlled 3 month study on vitamin & mineral supplements to assess the pre & post symptoms of ASD. According to this study, supplementation can be effectively used as an adjunct therapy for reducing the complications as these supplements are well tolerated by the ASD children.

## Essential Fatty Acids

Studies have reported that insufficient intake of essential fatty acids particularly omega 3 fatty acids has detrimental effects on the nervous system of ASD people, resulting in loss of concentration, hyperactivity, dyslexia, dyspraxia (Tsalamanio, 2006). Low levels of essential fatty acids in ASD is due to the enzyme defects which removes the essential fat from the brain cell membranes compared with the normal typically growing control groups (Bell et al., 2004). Supplementation of EPA & DHA & vitamin E (1.5g/day dosage) significantly improved speech & pronunciation among ASD children who were on investigation for 6 weeks along with the control groups. (Cohen et al.,2002).

## Probiotics

Probiotics increases the body's utilization of food components & essential vitamin synthesis along with impeding the development of harmful pathogens. Reports also indicate their various immuno-modulatory effects (Weichselbaum E, 2010). Due to the recurrent occurrence of the gastrointestinal dysfunction evident in ASD cases, use of probiotics has proven to exert a beneficial effect on restoring the normal gut flora & maintaining the associated complications (Crocen & Selvin et al., 2002).

## MINERALS

A comprehensive study by (Adams JB et al., 2011) found out that ASD children have lower levels of essential minerals (especially calcium, magnesium) and vitamins (B-complex) which was evident from their inadequate dietary intakes. (Latif et al., 2002) stated that iron deficiency is commonly linked with ASD children with low levels of serum ferritin, which could be due to insufficient intake of dietary iron. Iron deficiency during the developmental stage is associated with poor cognitive, motor, social functioning of the individual during his/her later years of life. A study by (Dosman et al., 2007) indicated that iron deficiency can cause sleep & nervous system disorders. Need for the screening of iron deficiency anemia was indicated in this study. Iron deficiency could be due to mal-absorption syndrome resulting from gastrointestinal symptoms. Therefore, supplementation with ferrous sulfate in iron deficient individuals has shown to significantly improve verbal learning and memory issues in ASD (Rossignol D.A., 2009) & also sleep disturbances.

Zinc deficiency is also implicated in ASD. Low levels of zinc in typically developing children are allied with learning problems, mental retardation & hyperactivity (Rossignol D.A., 2009). Another study by (Lei & Wang, et al., 2014) has indicated clinical depression with zinc deficiency. Lowered levels of zinc in RBC's by 40% constitute for the development of oxidative stress in ASD persons. On the contrary excess of zinc can aggravate the digestive function (McGinniset al., 2004).

## VITAMINS

ASD individuals generally have poor nutritional status, resulting in impaired digestion & intestinal inflammatory conditions that limit nutrient absorption. Due to these complications vital bacteria from the intestines gets depleted & therefore the production, absorption and availability of some vitamins are reduced. Many studies have been indicating promising results in restoring back the functioning of gut considerably in ASD cases with vitamin supplementations. Vitamin status biomarkers are employed to examine the possible association of them with the severity of ASD symptoms. Vitamin A is essential for the normal cell growth & differentiation particularly the epithelial cells lining the gut, brain etc. Supplementation of vitamin A (cod-liver oil; rich source) has been effective in treating the symptoms of autism where marked improvements were seen in language skills & maintaining eye contact (Megson, 2006). However, comprehensive clinical studies are required to confirm these findings.

(Kalueff et al., 2006) reported that Vitamin D has neuro-protective effect & also hinders the neurotransmitters interaction in the brain & hormones which can influence the patient behaviors. Another study by (Grant & Soles, 2009) examined the association of vitamin D deficiency posing a risk factor for the development of ASD in newborns in pregnant mothers. According to the findings mentioned above it is suggested that sufficient intake of vitamin D may reduce the risk of developing autism by supporting proper development of the brain & immune system.

Vitamin C is important for normal functioning of metabolic, antioxidant pathways & other co- enzymes for the synthesis of neurotransmitters. Deficiency of this vitamin is associated with dys-regulation of brain signaling glutamatergic system, associated with ASD's (Blaylock &Strunecka, 2009). It has been shown that vitamin C supplementation may be positively affecting the pathological behavior of ASD people (Adams & Holloway, 2004). From the above mentioned findings, it can be postulated that food/diet has a significant role in managing the symptoms of ASD and the possible benefits of it are as follows.

## Potential Benefits of Nutritional Interventions

- Improved alertness or 'being present'
- Improved speech & or usage of language & increase in effort to speak, number of words spoken, complexity of sentences & conversational speech.

- Improved social interactions including increased interest in peers & siblings, initiation of play, appropriate use of toys & improved tolerance in larger groups.
- Reduced self-stimulating & self-injurious behavior.
- Increased ability to focus & enhancement of cognitive function.
- Improved digestion, sleep & immune function.

## CONCLUSION

ASD is a multi-factorial disorder having a wide range of genetic and environmental causes. A sharp increase in the prevalence of ASD and increased difficulties in managing both physical & behavioral conditions has stimulated intense research around its potential factors and consequences so that curative & appropriate measures can be taken on time. Studies have provided extensive data on the dietary-related factors (nutritional deficiencies, gastrointestinal complications, food allergies) which could aggravate the symptoms. Studies also indicate gastrointestinal abnormalities, metabolic abnormalities, food allergies & sensitivities observed in ASD patients. Although numerous studies on the dietary problems have been studied globally, there is lack of literature among the Indian scenario. Nutrients are essential to regulate the biochemical processes in ASD people. Therefore, adequate nutritional status requires the consumption of nutrient dense food and proper digestion to breakdown and absorbs these foods. Dietary interventions should be substantiated with biochemical data which will benefit the ASD populations from timely and intensive interventions and in adulthood expand their options for living independently. Evidence has clearly shown that early intervention programs particularly nutritional approaches may yield a novel hope for efficiently managing the problems & treating ASD. Along with the intervention, parental involvement & support groups is very important. Therefore, this area of research warrants focused attention and effort.

## REFERENCES

American Psychiatric Association, (2013) *Diagnostic and Statistical Manual of Mental Disorders,* Fifth Edition. Arlington, VA: American Psychiatric Association.

Adams, J. B., & Holloway, C. (2004). Pilot study of a moderate dose multivitamin/mineral supplement for children with autistic spectrum disorder. *Journal of Alternative & Complementary Medicine*, *10*(6), 1033-1039.

Adams, J. B., Audhya, T., McDonough-Means, S., Rubin, R. A., Quig, D., Geis, E., & Barnhouse, S. (2011). Nutritional and metabolic status of children with autism vs. neurotypical children, and the association with autism severity. *Nutrition & metabolism*, 8(1), 34.

Autism and Developmental Disabilities Monitoring (ADDM) Network Centers for Disease Control and Prevention (CDC).

Bandini, L. G., Anderson, S. E., Curtin, C., Cermak, S., Evans, E. W., Scampini, R., et al. (2010). Food selectivity in children with autism spectrum disorders and typically developing children. *Journal of Pediatrics*, 157, 259-264.

Bell, J. G., MacKinlay, E. E., Dick, J. R., MacDonald, D. J., Boyle, R. M., & Glen, A. C. A. (2004). Essential fatty acids and phospholipase A 2 in autistic spectrum disorders. *Prostaglandins, Leukotrienes and Essential Fatty Acids,* 71(4), 201-204.

Barr, S. I., Murphy, S. P., Poos, M. I., (2002). *Interpreting and using the dietary references intakes in dietary assessment of individuals and groups*, 102(6):780-8.

Blaylock, R. L., & Strunecka, A. (2009). Immune-glutamatergic dysfunction as a central mechanism of the autism spectrum disorders. *Current medicinalchemistry,* 16(2), 157-170.

Cornish, E. (1998). A balanced approach toward healthy eating in autism. *Journal of Human Nutrition &Dietetics,* 11, 501-509.

Croen, L. A., Grether, J. K., & Selvin, S. (2002). Descriptive epidemiology of autism in a California population: who is at risk? *Journal of autism and developmentaldisorders,* 32(3), 217-224.

Dosman, C. F., Brian, J. A., Drmic, I. E., Senthilselvan, A., Harford, M. M., Smith, R. W., & Roberts, S. W. (2007). Children with autism: effect of iron supplementation on sleep and ferritin. *Pediatric neurology*, 36(3), 152-158.

Elder, J. H. (2008). The gluten-free, casein-free diet in autism: an overview with clinical implications. *Nutrition in Clinical Practice*, 23(6), 583-588

Emond, A., Emmett, P., Steer, C., & Golding, J. (2010).Feeding symptoms, dietary patterns, and growth in young children with autism spectrum disorders. *Pediatrics, 126*, e337–e342.

Feingold, S. M., Molitoris, D., Song, Y., Liu, C., Vaisanen, M. L., Bolte, E., & Collins, M. D. (2002). Gastrointestinal microflora studies in late-onset autism. *Clinical Infectious Diseases, 35*(Supplement1), 6–16.

Feingold, B. F. (1975). Hyperkinesis and learning disabilities linked to artificial food flavors and colors. *AJN The American Journal of Nursing*, 75(5), 797-803.

Grant, W. B., & Soles, C. M. (2009). Epidemiologic evidence for supporting the role of maternal vitamin D deficiency as a risk factor for the development of infantile autism. *Dermato-endocrinology,* 1(4), 223-228.

Gottschall E. (2004) Digestion-gut-autism connection: the specific carbohydrate diet. *Med. Veritas*, 1, 261-271.

Herndon, A. C., DiGuiseppi, C., Johnson, S., Leiferman, J., Reynolds, A. (2009). Does nutritional intake differ between children with autism spectrum disorders and children with typical development? *Journal of Autismand Developmental Disorders*, 39, 212-222.

Ho, H. H., Eaves, L. C., & Peabody, D. (1997). Nutrient intake and obesity in children with autism. *Focus on Autism and Other Developmental Disabilities,* 12, 187-193.

Hediger, M. L., England, L. J., Molloy, C. A., Yu, K. F., Manning-Courtney, P., & Mills, J. L. (2008). Reduced bone cortical thickness in boys with autism or autism spectrum disorder. *Journal of Autism and Developmental Disorders*, 38, 848-856.

Howlin, P. & Moore, A. (1997) *Diagnosis in autism: a survey of 1200 patients in the UK*, autism 1: 135-162. Google scholar.

Jepson B., Johnson J. (2007) *Changing the course of autism: A scientific approach for parents and physicians*. 1st edn, Sentient Publications Boulder. ISBN-10: 1591810612.

James B., Adams, Tapan Audhya, Sharon McDonough-Means, Robert A. Rubin, David Quig, Elizabeth Geis, Eva Gehn, *Effect of a vitamin/mineral supplement on children and adults with autism* Published online Dec 12, 2011.

Johnson, C. R., Handen, B. L., Mayer-Costa, M., & Sacco, K. (2008). Eating habits and dietary status in young children with autism. *Journal of Developmental andPhysical Disabilities*, 20, 437-448.

Kalueff, A. V., Minasyan, A., Keisala, T., Kuuslahti, M., Miettinen, S., &Tuohimaa, P. (2006). The vitamin D neuroendocrine system as a target for novel neurotropic drugs. *CNS & Neurological Disorders-Drug Targets* (Formerly *Current Drug Targets-CNS & Neurological Disorders*), 5(3), 363-371.

Klin, A., Jones, W., Schultz, R., Volkmar, F., & Cohen, D., (2002). Defining and quantifying the social phenotype in autism. *American Journal of Psychiatry*, 159(6), 895-908.

Latif A., et al., Iron Deficiency in Autism and Asperger Syndrome. *Autism* 2002, 6:103.

Levy, S., Souders, M. C., Ittenbach, R. F., Giarelli, E., Mulberg, A., & Pinto-Martin, J. (2007). Relationship of dietary intake to gastrointestinal symptoms in children with autistic spectrum disorders. *Biological Psychiatry*, 61, 492–497.

Ledford, J. R., &Gast, D. L. (2006). Feeding problems in children with autism spectrum disorders: A review. *Focus on Autism and Other Developmental Disabilities, 21*(3), 153–166.

Li, S. O., Wang, J. L., Bjørklund, G., Zhao, W. N., & Yin, C. H. (2014). Serum copper and zinc levels in individuals with autism spectrum disorders. *Neuroreport*, 25(15), 1216-1220.

Lindsay, R. L., Arnold, L. E., Aman, M. G., Vitiello, B., Posey, D. J., McDougle, C. J., et al. (2006). Dietary status and impact of risperidone on nutritional balance in children with autism: a pilot study. *Journal of Intellectual and Developmental Disability*, 31, 204-209.

Lucarelli S., Frediani T., Zingoni A. M., et al. (1995) Food allergy and infantile autism. *Panminerva Med* 37, 137–141.

Matson, J. L., & Fodstad, J. C. (2009). The treatment of food selectivity and other feeding problems in children with autism spectrum disorders. *Research in Autism Spectrum Disorders, 3*, 455–461.

Megson, M. N. (2000). Is autism a G-alpha protein defect reversible with natural vitamin A? *Medical hypotheses,* 54(6), 979-983.

McGinnis, W. R. (2004). Oxidative stress in autism. *Alternative therapies in health and medicine,* 10(6), 22-36.

Marí-Bauset, S., Llopis-González, A., Zazpe-García, I., Marí-Sanchis, A., & Morales-Suárez-Varela, M. (2015). Nutritional status of children with autism spectrum disorders (ASDs): A case–control study. *Journal of Autism and Developmental Disorders, 45*(1), 203–212.

Pauling, L. (1968). Orthomolecular psychiatry. *Science*, 160(825), 265-271.

Purkayastha, M., Girimaji, S., Srinath, S., & Sheshadri, S. P. (1997). Clinical profile in mental retardation. *Research endeavors in child and adolescent psychiatry in India.* Goa: IACAM, 48-53.

Raiten, D. J., & Massaro, T. (1986). Perspectives on the nutritional ecology of autistic children. *Journal of Autism and Developmental Disorders,* 16(2), 133-143.

Rossignol, D. A. (2009). Novel and emerging treatments for autism spectrum disorders: a systematic review. *Ann Clin Psychiatry*, 21(4), 213-36.

Russell, P. S., Daniel, A., Russell, S., Mammen, P., Abel, J. S., Raj, L. E., & Thomas, N. (2010). Diagnostic accuracy, reliability and validity of Childhood Autism Rating Scale in India. *World Journal of Pediatrics*, 6(2), 141-147.

Sabra A., Bellanti J. A., Hartmann D., et al. (2012) Gastrointestinal and behavioral dysfunction in children with non-IgE mediated food allergy, ileal-nodular-lymphoid hyperplasia (ILNH) and low Th1 function: a new clinical-immunologicconstellation. *J Food Allergy* 1, 36–43.

Siegel, B. (1997) 'Coping with the Diagnosis of Autism', in D. J. Cohen & F.R. Volkmar (eds.) *Handbook of Autism and Pervasive Developmental Disorders.* New York: Wiley. Google Scholar.

Schmitt, L., Heiss, C. J., & Campbell, E. E. (2008). A comparison of nutrient intake and eating behavior of boys with and without autism. *Topics in Clinical Nutrition,* 23, 23-31.

Shearer, T. R., Larson, K., Neuschwander, J., & Gedney, B. (1982). Minerals in the hair and nutrient intake of autistic children. *Journal of Autism and DevelopmentalDisorders*, 12, 25-34.

Sowmyanath (2014). *Feeding problems in children with autism interactive autism network.* Baltimore: Kennedy Krieger Institute.

Srinath, S., Chowdhury, J., Bhide, A. V., Narayanan, H. S., Shivaprakash, Z. Z. (1989). Descriptive study of infantile autism. *Nimhans Journal,* 7(1), 77-81.

Tsalamanios, E., Yanni, A. E., & Koutsari, C. (2006). Omega-3 fatty acids: Role in the prevention and treatment of psychiatric disorders. *Current Psychiatry Reviews,* 2(2), 215-234.

Valenci-McDermott M., McVicar K., Rapin I., et al. (2006) Frequency of gastrointestinal symptoms in children with autistic spectrum disorders and association with family history of autoimmune disease. *J Dev Behav Pediatr* 27, 128–136.

Wei, X., Yanjuan, Z., Caihong, S., Jia, W., & Lijie W. (2010). A preliminary study on nutritional status and intake in Chinese children with autism. *EuropeanJournal of Pediatrics*, e-published ahead of print.

Weichselbaum, E. (2010). Potential benefits of probiotics– main findings of an in-depth review. *Br J Community Nurs,* 15(3), 110-112.

Wheeler, J. J., Baggett, B. A., Fox, J., & Blevins, L. (2006). Treatment integrity: A review of intervention studies conducted with children with autism. *Focus on Autismand Other Developmental Disabilities*, 21(1), 45-54.

Zimmer M H, Hart L C, Courtney P M, Murray D S, Bing N M, Summer S.(2012) Food variety as a predictor of nutritional status among children with autism. *J Autism Dev Disord*; 42:549-556.

## BIOGRAPHICAL SKETCHES

### *Seema Siddiqi*

**Affiliation:** University of Mysore

**Education:** MSc in Food Science and Nutrition

**Research and Professional Experience:** Currently pursuing PhD in Food science and nutrition from University of Mysore. Basically working on autism.

**Professional Appointments:** seema_siddiqi@yahoo.com

**Honors:** awarded best paper presentation at International conference on millets at Periyar University Salem, India on January 9-10 2020.

**Publications from the Last 3 Years:**

1) Seema Siddiqi, Asna Urooj & Melwin James D'Souza, "Dietary Patterns and Anthropometric Measures of Indian Children with Autism Spectrum Disorder," *Journal of Autism and Developmental Disorders,* Vol 43(09) December 2018.doi.org/10.1007/s10803-018-3850-0.
2) Satish Anandan, Seema Siddiqi, Syeda Farha Siraj and Urooj Asna, Protective Effect of Apigenin from *Morusindica.*L against Methylglyoxal Induced Oxidative DNA Damage, *Int J Pharm Biol Sci.*DOI: https://doi.org/10.21276/ijpbs.2019.9.2.24.
3) Asna Urooj and Seema Siddiqi. Analytical and nutritional implications of carbohydrate digestibility with special reference to *Indian foods in Food Chemistry*. New Delhi Publishers, India 2018.
4) Seema Siddiqi, Lakshmi S and Asna Urooj. Iron bio-accessibility and nutritional attributes of selected disease specific formulations. *Def. Life Sci. J;* 2017:2(2)1-6, DOI : 10.14429/dlsj.2.

### *Asna Urooj*

**Affiliation:** University of Mysore

**Education:** PhD in Food Science and Nutrition

**Research and Professional Experience:** since 1987 on diabetes, CVD, Clinical nutrition, Autsim

**Professional Appointments:** asnau321@gmail.comasnaurooj@foodsci.uni-mysore.ac.in.

**Honors:**

1) Dr. Rajammal P Devadas Memorial Award- for outstanding contributions in the field of applied Nutritional Sciences for 2017, by Nutrition Society of India.
2) Academician Award – By Nutritionists Republic for highest publications by a Nutritionist in 2013.
3) Prof G.S. Bains lifetime achievement award –for credible achievement in the area of Nutrition for the year 2011, by Association of Food Scientist's & Technologists, India.
4) State Award – Dr Kalpana Chawla award for young women scientist in the field of Science & Technology for the year 2009 by Government of Karnataka.
5) Young scientist award- Indian Dietetic Association, Nutrition Society of India, RSSDI, International College of Nutrition.
6) 40 best research paper awards in various national and international conferences.

**Publications from the Last 3 Years:**

1) Sheetal.V.Shenoy, Sudha Sairam, Namratha Pai K and Asna Urooj. Socio-demographic, anthropometric and biochemical profile of subjects

with head and neck cancer: a pilot study. *British J Medical & Health Research,* 2017, 4 (6), 44-54.

2) Charlotte G. K. and Asna Urooj. Obesity status and lifestyle pattern of pre and post Menopausal urban - employed women of Mysore city, India. *Advances in Obesity, Weight Management & Control* 2017, 6(2): 00148, 1-11. DOI: 10.15406/aowmc.2017.06.00148.
3) Vanitha Reddy, Asna Urooj, Sudha S., Faiyaz Ahmed and N. N. Prasad. Hypocholesterolemic effect of Moringaoleifera polyphenols in rats fed with high fat and cholesterol diet. *Malaysian J Nutrition2017,* 23(2): 473 – 478.
4) Seema Siddiqi, Lakshmi S. and Asna Urooj. Iron bio-accessibility and nutritional attributes of selected disease specific formulations. *Def. Life Sci. J;* 2017: 2(2)1-6, DOI : 10.14429/dlsj.2.
5) Sowmya Rajshekhar and Asna Urooj. Significance of Inflammatory biomarkers in detecting Risk for CVD in type 2 diabetic subjects. *Journal of Indian Dietetic Association.* 2017, 39(2): 21-32.
6) Bhagirathi L & Asna Urooj. Nutritional Assay and Organoleptic Evaluation of the Cashew apple in Coastal Karnataka," *Trends in Bio Sciences,* 2017, 10(1):415-418.
7) Bhagirathi L and Asna Urooj. "Processing Technology for utilization of cashew apple (Anacardium occidental L)," *Indian Food Industry 2017.*
8) Sheetal. Vijayakumar Shenoy, Sudha Sairam, Namratha Pai Kotebagilu and Asna Urooj. "Socio-demographic, anthropometric and biochemical profile of subjects with Head and neck cancer: A pilot study" *British J Medical and Health Research 2017*; 4 (6), 44-54.
9) Supriya. S., Asna Urooj and Krishnakanth. T.P. Inhibition of platelet aggregation and antioxidative effect of some plant foods. *Eur J Biomedical and Pharmaceutical Sciences.* 2017 4 (8):731-740.
10) Lawrence T.Mugambi, Sudha Sairam, Linda Grace Roy and Asna Urooj. "Nutritional Status of University Graduates Sports Students," *Journal of Indian Dietetic Association*, 2017, 40(1), pp.40 - 47.
11) Chandan Vinay Srigiripura, Asna Urooj, Chaya SindaghattaKrishnarao, Mahesh AnandPadukudru. Validation of Fat-Free Mass Estimation Using Prediction Equations in Male Patients with Chronic Obstructive

Pulmonary Disease. *International Journal of Nutrition, Pharmacology, Neurological Diseases,* 2017, 7(4): 94-100.

12) Anandan, S., Kotebagilu, N.P., Shivanna, L.M. and Urooj, A. Inhibitory potency of C-glycosyl flavonoids from morus sp. on advanced glycation end products. *Journal of Biologically Active Products from Nature,* 2017, 7(5), pp.391-400.
13) Asna Urooj and Vishalakshi Devi D. *Asian Journal of Phytomedicine and Clinical Research.* 5(2), 2017, 67-75.
14) Lohith Mysuru Shivanna, Namratha Pai Kotebagilu and Asna Urooj. Validation of assessment categories of the Patient Generated-Subjective Global Assessment tool in classifying the nutritional status of cancer patients. *International Journal of Nutrition, Pharmacology, Neurological Diseases,* 2018; 8:79-85.
15) Naveen Y.P., DivyaRupini, Faiyaz Ahmed and Asna Urooj. In vitro Hypoglycemic Potential of Spices; Cinnamon and Cumin. *Pakistan J Pharmaceutical Sciences,* 2018, 30 (6). (0.581) 5x =2.90
16) Satish Anandan, Syeda Farha S., Mahadeva M. J. and Asna Urooj Glucosinolates and antioxidant properties of Brassica oleracea var. capitata.*Food Science and Nutrition Technology 2018; 3 (3) :000152.*
17) Vanitha Reddy and Asna Urooj. In vitro bile acid sequestering properties of Morusindica L leaves. *Annal of Phytomedicine* 2018 7(1): 96-100.
18) Namratha Pai K., Lohith M. S., Asna Urooj, Anil Thomas, Mukesh S., Sathya M.Socio-Demographic, Somatic and Disease Profile of Cancer Patients in Tertiary Care Centres of a City in Karnataka, *Int J Med Public Health.* 2018;8(2):82-8.
19) Ranjini T.R. and Asna Urooj. Changes in oxidative and antioxidant status in acute Myocardial infarct patients. *Br J Med Health Res.* 2018; 5(07).
20) Satish Anandan, Syeda Farha S. and Asna Urooj. Quantification of flavonoids by UPLC-MS and its antibacterial activity from Brassica oleraceavar. CapitataL. *GSC Biological and Pharmaceutical Sciences,* 2018, 05(01), 109–114.

21) Asna Urooj, Florence Suma and Ritika Kalra. In vitro bio-accessibility of calcium from eggshell powder and calcium salts. *J Advances in Food Science and Technology,* 2018 5(3): 72-80.
22) Kaneez Haleema, Chandan Vinay and Asna Urooj. Evaluation of popped euryaleferoxseeds as a potent functional food based on its nutritional profile, functional attributes and macronutrient digestibility. *Advances in Food Science and Technology.* 2018, 5(3): 81-87.
23) Asna Urooj and Seema Siddiqi. Analytical and nutritional implications of carbohydrate digestibility with special reference to Indian foods in *Food Chemistry*. New Delhi Publishers, India 2018.

# INDEX

## A

## B



## C

## D

## H



## I

## S



## T